CONTENTS

Section A: Basic Wound Principle

Chapter 1 Clinical Applied Anatomy in Wound Care... 2

Chapter 2 Definition and Classification of Wound, and Stages of Wound Healing.... 6

Chapter 3 Wound Assessment and Documentation... 13

Chapter 4 Wound Infection and Bacteriology in Wound Care.................................. 19

Chapter 5 Nutrition in Wound Care... 27

Chapter 6 Principle of Wound Closure.. 37

Section B: Concept of Wound Care Management

Chapter 7 Management of Acute Wound
 a) Burn Wound.. 54
 b) Traumatic Wound... 60

Chapter 8 Management of Chronic Wound
 a) Diabetic Foot ulcer... 67
 b) Venous Ulcer... 77
 c) Arterial Ulcer... 83
 d) Pressure Ulcer... 90

Chapter 9 Management of Non-Healing Ulcer.. 98

Chapter 10 Management of Life Threatening Wound................................. 106

Chapter 11 Analgesia for Wound Dressing Related Procedures................. 113

Section C: Practical Aspect of Wound Care

Chapter 12 Standard Operating Procedure on Wound Dressing............................ 124

Chapter 13 Wound Cleansing.. 129

Chapter 14 Type of Dressing... 132

Chapter 15 Wound Debridement.. 137

Chapter 16 Adjunctive Treatment
    a) Honey Treatment... 146
    b) Hyperbaric Oxygen Therapy.................................. 152
    c) Negative Pressure Wound Therapy (NPWT)......... 157

Chapter 17 Algorithm for Wound Care Treatment................................... 163

Appendix.. 168

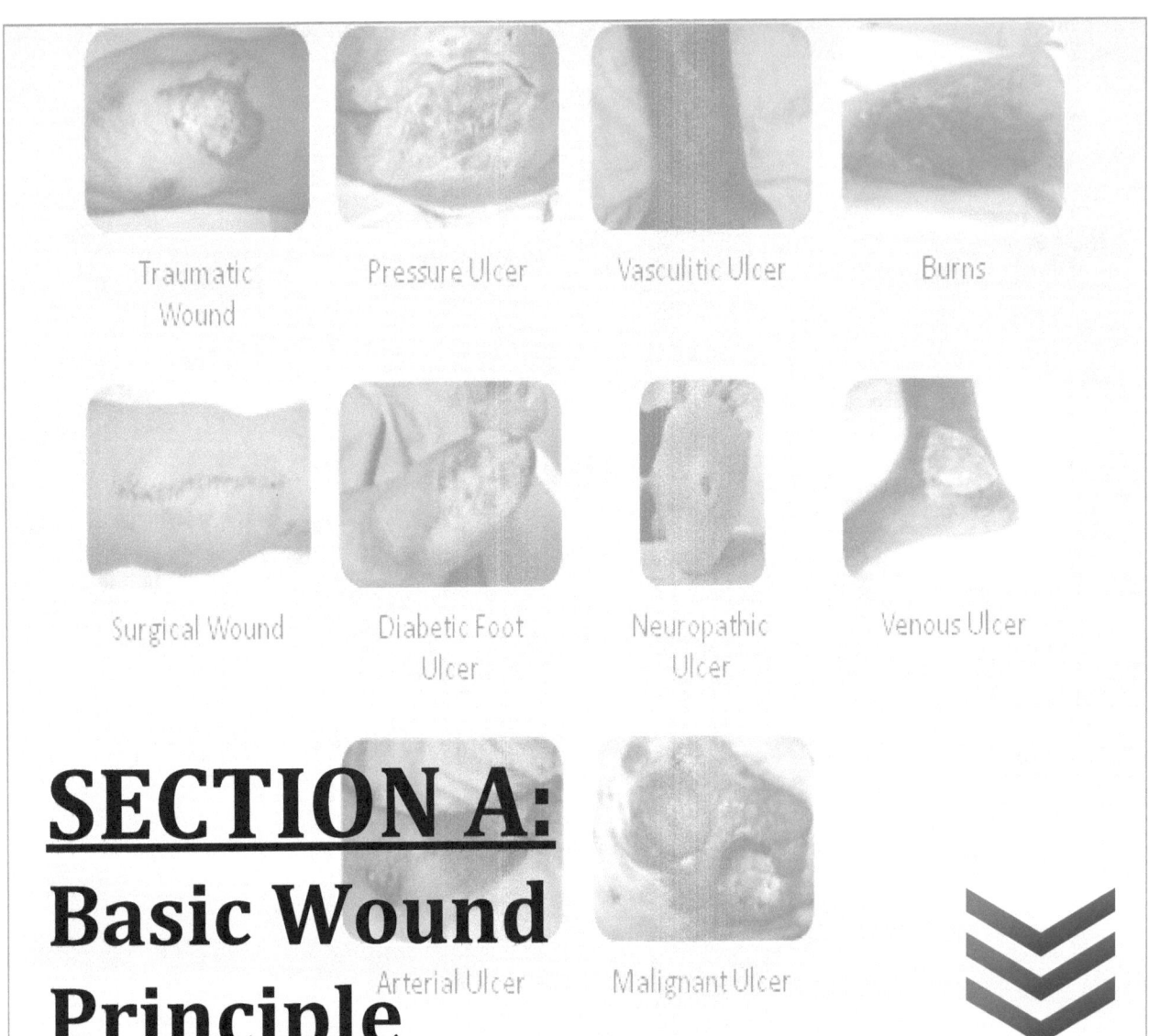

SECTION A: Basic Wound Principle

CHAPTER	TOPIC	CONTRIBUTORS
Chapter 1	Clinical Applied Anatomy in Wound Care	Dr Mohd Farid
Chapter 2	Definition and Classification of Wound, and Stages of Wound Healing	Dr Haris Ali Dr Mohammad Anwar Hau
Chapter 3	Wound Assessment and Documentation	Dr Harikrishna K.R Nair
Chapter 4	Wound Infection and Bacteriology in Wound Care	Dr Nurahan Maning
Chapter 5	Nutrition in Wound Care	Puan Mageswary Puan Harizah Puan Nurul Huda
Chapter 6	Principle of Wound Closure	Dr Normala

CHAPTER 1: Clinical Applied Anatomy in Wound Care

1-1. What is the Skin?

- Skin is the outer covering of the body and thus provides protection.

- It is the largest organ in our body in term of weight and surface areas.

- Its thickness ranges from 0.5 to 4.0 mm depending on location.

- It consists of different tissues that are joined together to perform several essential functions.

- It is a dynamic organ in a constant of change; whereby the outer layers are continuously shed and replaced by the inner cells moving to the surface.

- Structurally, the skin consists of 3 principal layers.

    - Epidermis: outer most layer, thinner portion, composed of epithelium.

    - Dermis: middle layer, thicker, consists of connective tissue.

    - Subcutaneous: deepest layer, also known as superficial fascia or hypodermis; consists of areola and adipose tissues.

    - Fibers from the dermis extend down into the subcutaneous layer and anchor the skin to it.

    - The subcutaneous layer, in turn, attaches to underlying tissues and organs.

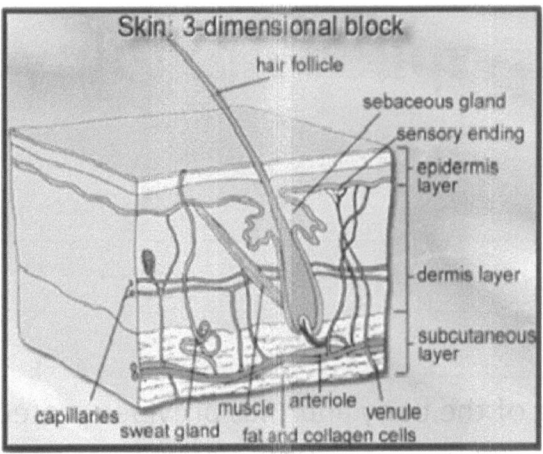

Figure 1.1 Layers of the skin

1-2. Function of the Skin

a. Body temperature regulation
b. Protection
c. Sensation
d. Excretion
e. Immune function
f. Blood reservoir
g. Synthesis of Vitamin D

1-3. Epidermis

- Epidermis is avascular labile tissue which continuously regenerates.

- It receives nutrients from the dermis below

- Comprised of stratified squamous epithelium and contains four principal types of cells.

    i) ***Keratinocytes***- produce proinflammatory mediators, participate in wound healing, and contribute in ultraviolet radiation protection.

    ii) ***Melanocytes:*** modulate skin colour through melanogenesis (melanin production).

    iii) ***Langerhan Cell:*** role in immune response to pathogens

    iv) ***Meckel's Cell:*** " touch cells"- responsible to sensation

1-4. Dermis

- The second principal layer of skin.

- Composed of connective tissue containing collagen, elastic fibers which provides strength, extensibility, and elasticity.

- Thickness depending on the anatomical site (e.g. very thick in the palms and soles and very thin in the eyelids, penis, and scrotum)

- Contains nerves, glands, hair follicles and also receptors for heart, cold, pain, pressure, itch and tickle.

- It has rich blood supply from vascular plexus in the deep dermis. Through extensive vascular network (ascending arterioles and capillary loops), the blood supply eventually reaches upper layers of dermis

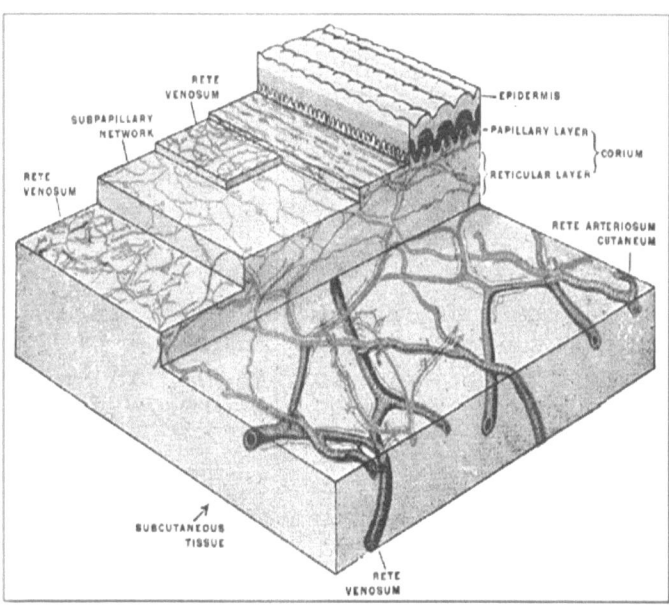

Figure 1.2 Blood supply of the skin

1-5. Subcutaneous layer

- The deepest layer of skin, also known as **subcutis** or hypodermis

- It varies in thickness and depth.

- Comprised of adipose tissue, connective tissue and blood vessels. Forms a network of **collagen** and **fat cells**.

- Responsible for conserving the body's heat and protects body organs from pressure injury

1-6. Skin and Wound

- Superficial wound that damage the epithelium only, can heal by epithelial regeneration (reconstitute) and may have little scar formation.

- Deeper wound; incisional and excisional skin wounds that damage the dermis will heal through the formation of a collagen scar.

- Regeneration requires an intact connective tissue scaffold.

- Scar formation occur if the extracellular matrix framework is damaged, causing alteration of the tissue architecture.

- Epidermal appendages do not regenerate and there remains as connective tissue scar.

Points to Remember:

- Blood supply is essential in wound healing
- Blood supply is predominantly found in the dermis

Reference

1. Harold Ellis. Clinical Anatomy : A revision and applied anatomy for clinical students, Tenth Edition

2. Henry Gray. ANATOMY, DESCRIPTIVE AND SURGICAL, 1901 EDITION

3. Anne M.R.Agur, Ming J.Lee . Grants Atlas of anatomy Tenth Edition, LIPPINCOT WILLIAM & WILKINS

4. Kenneth S.Saladin, Leslie Miller. Anatomy & Physiology The Unity of Form and Function , Tenth edition

Chapter 2: Definition and Classification of Wound, and Stages of Wound Healing

2-1. Definition

Wound A wound is an injury to the integument or to the underlying structures;
It is visible result of individual cell death or damage; that may or may not result in a loss of skin integrity whereby physiological function of the tissue is impaired.

Ulcer An interruption of continuity of an epithelial surface with an inflamed base.
It is usually a *result of an underlying or internal etiology.*

2-2. Classification of Wound

There is no standard classification of wound. The classification used in this guideline is based on:

(A) Timing:
- **Acute**: sudden disruption of skin integrity; usually due to trauma or surgery
- **Chronic**: wound that failed to proceed through an orderly and timely process to produce anatomic and functional integrity
- **Non-healing wound**: Any wound that has no signs of healing process within 2 to 4 weeks after appropriate intervention.

(B) Etiology: refer Figure 2.1

2-3. Etiology of Wound

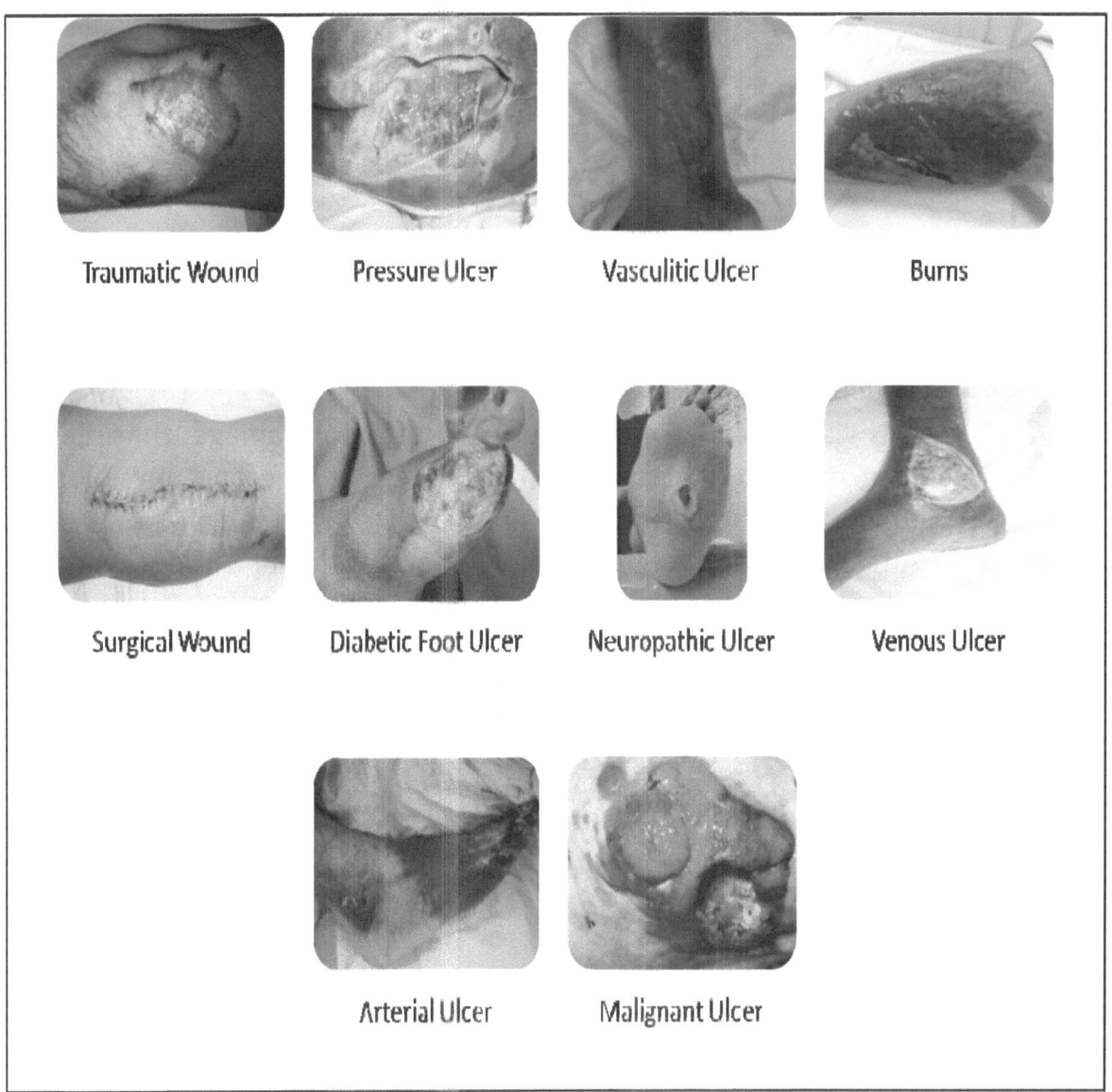

Figure 2.1 Different etiology of wound

2-4. Wound Healing

Definition:

Wound healing is a complex series of reactions and interactions among cells and "mediators" in four distinct and overlapping phases.

Phases of wound healing:

Wound undergoes 4 phases of healing:
1. Haemostasis
2. Inflammation (0-3 days)
3. Proliferation (3-24 days)
4. Maturation (24 – 365 days)

As shown in Figure 2.2 and Table 2.1

Type of wound healing:

Wound healing by primary intention:

1. Primary healing: when a clean surgical/traumatic wound is closed primarily; healing with minimal scar formation.
2. Delayed primary healing: closure of wound 3-5 days after the initial debridement and dressing of the wound (before granulation tissue formation).

Wound healing by secondary intention:

Secondary healing: When there is extensive tissue loss with inability to oppose edges. Healing is with granulation, contraction and re-epithelialisation; resulting in scar formation.

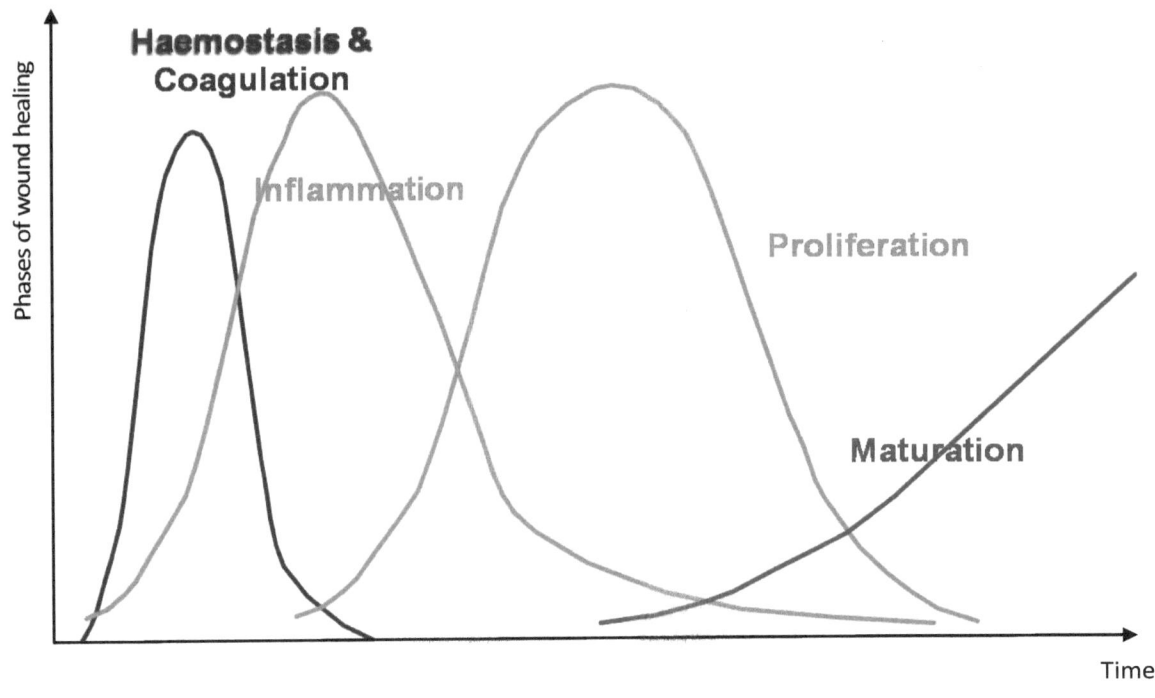

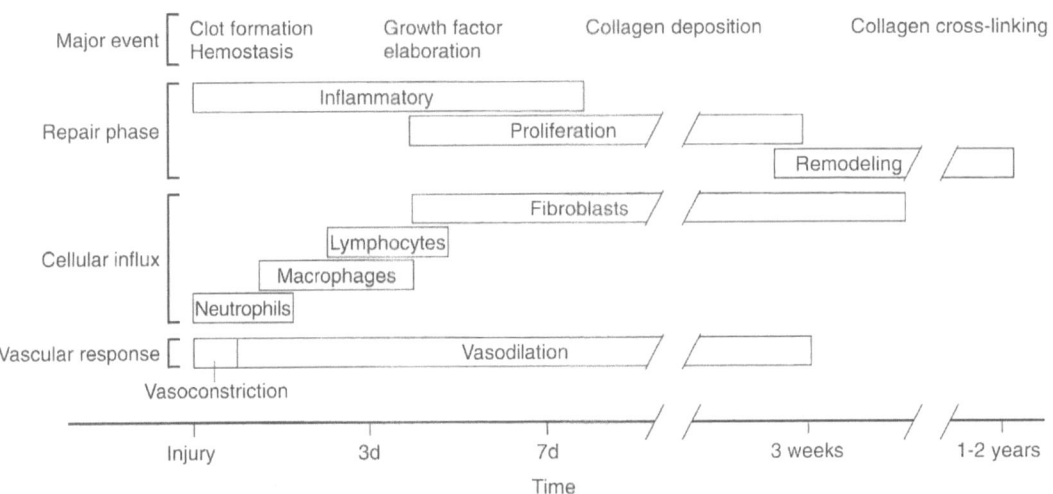

Figure 2.2 Summary on phases of wound healing

SECTION A: BASIC WOUND PRINCIPLE | 9

Table 2.1 Phases of wound healing

Phases	Haemostasis	Inflammation	Proliferation	Maturation
Time	Immediate	Day 1-3	Day 2 – Week 3	1 Week – several weeks
Key cells	Platelets	Neutrophils Macrophages	Fibroblast	
Process involved	<ul><li>Vasoconstriction</li><li>Platelet adhesion and degranulation</li><li>Platelet aggregation</li><li>Activation of coagulation cascade</li></ul>	<ul><li>Vasodilatation</li><li>Activation of complement cascade</li><li>Infiltration of wound with neutrophils and monocytes</li><li>Phagocytosis of bacteria, foreign body and cells debris</li></ul>	<ul><li>Fibroblast migration</li><li>Reconstitution of dermis - Fibroplasia - Angiogenesis</li><li>Re-ephitelialization</li><li>Wound contraction</li></ul>	<ul><li>Collagen degradation (type III)</li><li>Collagen synthesis (type I)</li></ul>
Outcome	Fibrin clot	Healthy wound bed	<ul><li>Granulation tissue</li><li>New epithelium</li><li>Contracted wound</li></ul>	Increased tissue strength

2-5. Factors Affecting Wound Healing

1. *Local Factors*
    - Tissue oxygenation
    - Infection
    - Foreign body
    - Venous insufficiency

2. *Systemic Factors*
    - Advancing age
    - Obesity
    - Ischaemia
    - Malnutrition
    - Disease: Diabetes, Anaemia,

- Medications: Glucocorticoid steroids, NSAIDs, Chemotherapy
- Alcohol and smoking
- Immuno-deficiency: Cancer, radiation therapy, AIDS

2-6. Clinical Features of Wound Healing

Normal phases of wound healing

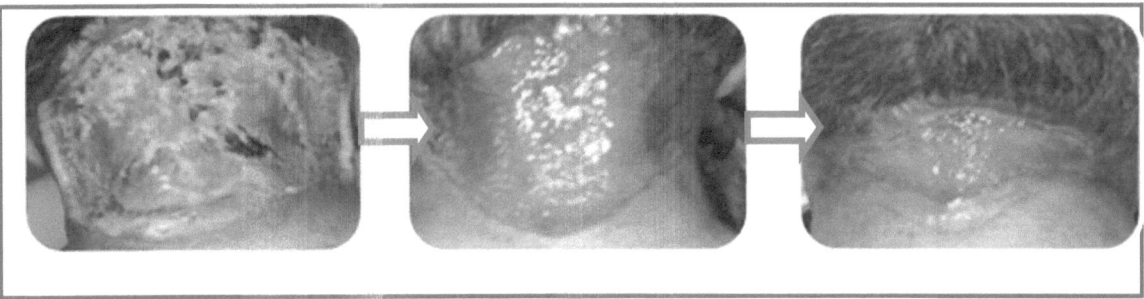

Figure 2.3 Normal progression of wound healing

Non-healing wound

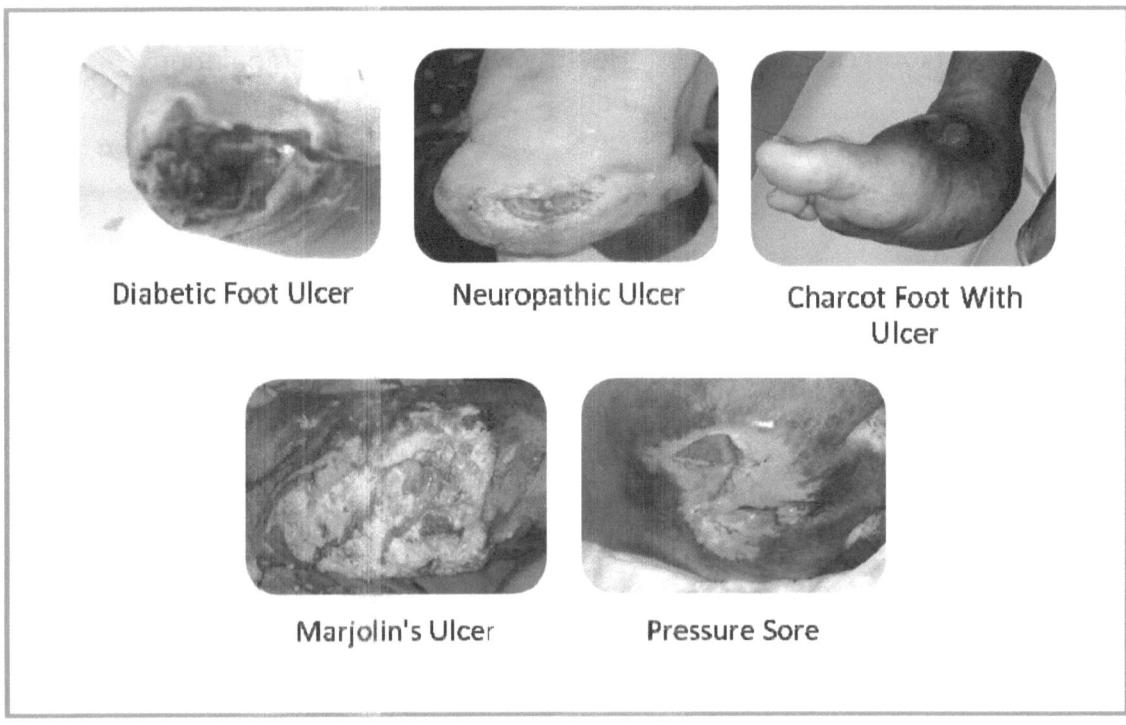

Figure 2.4 Picture of non-healing wound

Point to Remember:

- To understand the different stages and factors involved in normal physiology of wound healing.

Reference

1. Hermans MH. Wounds and Ulcers: Back to the old nomenclature. Wounds Volume 22, Issue 11, November 2010, page 289-293.

2. Enoch S, Leaper DJ. Basic science of wound healing. Surgery (Oxford), 2008, 26:2:31-37

3. Li J, Chen J, Kirsner R. Pathophysiology of acute wound healing. Clinics in Dermatology, 2007,25:9-18

4. Lazarus et al Arch Dermatol. 1994, 130 (4): 489-93

CHAPTER 3

Wound Assessment and Documentation

Dr. Harikrishna K.R Nair

3-1. Wound Assessment

General assessment:

The general assessment is to identify and eliminate any underlying causes or contributing factors which may impede the wound healing process; the causes include:

- Age (extremes of age)
- Diseases or co morbidities (e.g. diabetes mellitus , renal impairment)
- Medication (steroids , chemotherapy)
- Obesity
- Nutrition (refer to chapter on nutrition)
- Impaired blood supply (refer to chapter on arterial and venous ulcers)
- Lifestyle (smoking , alcohol)

Local wound assessment (Figure 3.1):

Local assessment is an ongoing process and should include:

- A review of the wound history (How, What, When, Where, Who)
- Assessment of the physical wound characteristics
    - location, size, base/depth
    - presence of pain
    - condition of the wound bed

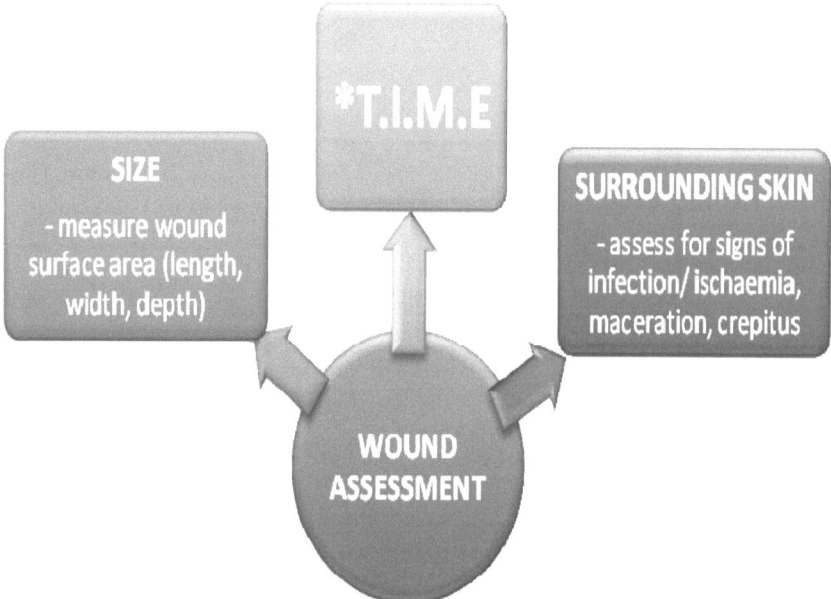

Figure 3.1 Local wound assessment

T.I.M.E. - Principles of Wound Bed Assessment and Preparation:

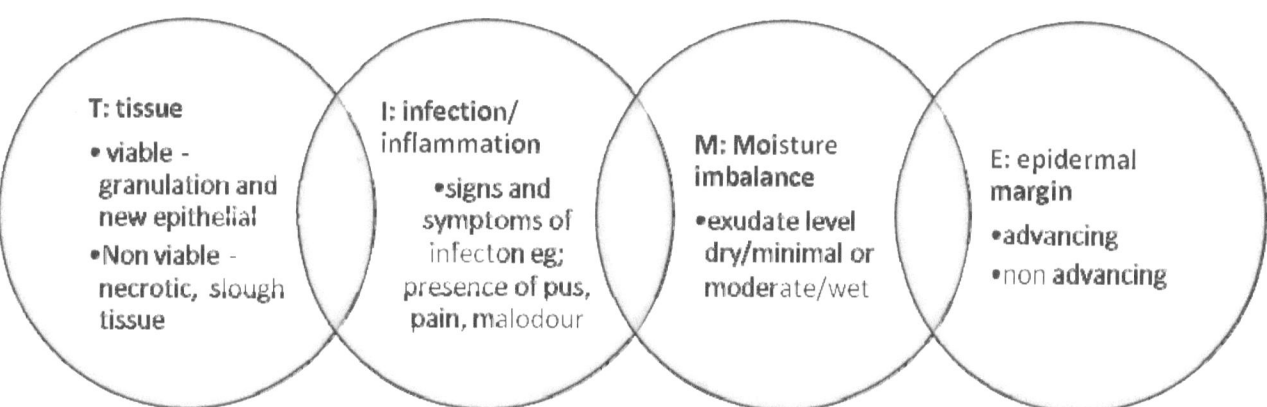

Clinical Appearance:

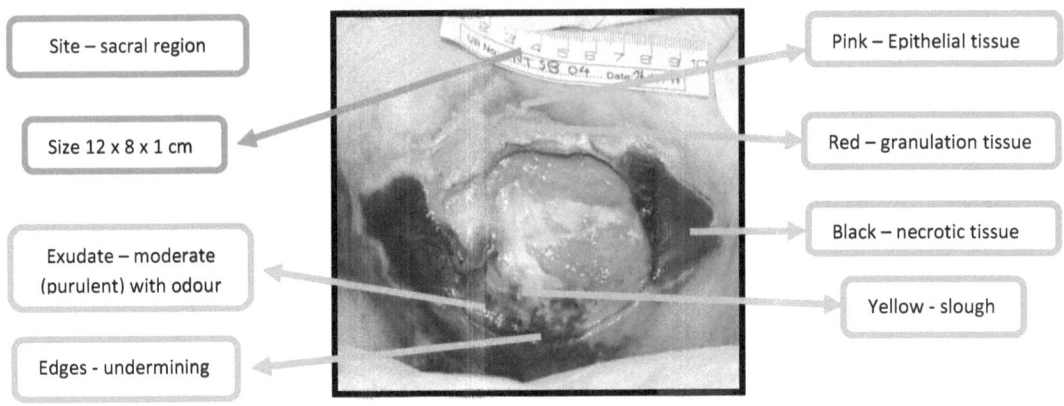

Figure 3.2 Stage 3 pressure ulcer

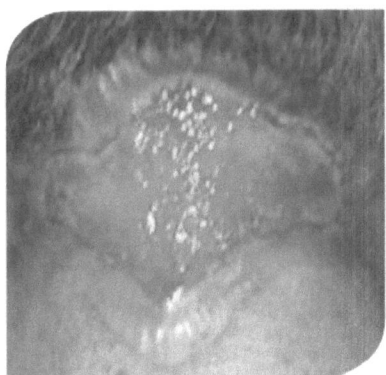

Figure 3.3 Advancing epidermal margin (epithelialisation)

3-2. Wound Documentation

Aim of Documentation
- Record the history
- Identify etiological factors
- Identify intrinsic and extrinsic factors that may affect wound healing
- Obtain a baseline for future comparison
- Provide a legal and organizational record
- Use in evaluation and planning of wound management
- Monitor wound progress
- Communication tool

Principles of Documentation

- Timely, Accurate and objective
- Concise and Comprehensive
- Legible writing, Include signature and printed name
- Use only organizationally approved abbreviations and colloquialisms
- Regular, Systematic, Standardized, Easily interpreted And Time efficient
- Used to inform management decisions

The findings of wound assessment and the dressing solution / material should be documented in wound chart as in figure 3.4 .

Point to Remember:

- Wound assessment includes systemic and local assessment.
- T.I.M.E principle
- Wound documentation according to Wound Chart as in Appendix 1

Reference

1. TIME concept

2. Dr. Gary Sibbald, et al. Preparing the wound bed for healing- debridement, bacterial balance & moisture balance. Ostomy/ wound management, 2000, 46(1)

3. Falanga V. Wound Repair Regen 2000, 8(5):347-52

Chapter 4: Wound Infection and Bacteriology in Wound Care

Dr. Nurahan Maning

4-1. Pathway of Wound Infection

CONTAMINATION
Presence of microorganisms that do not multiply or cause clinical problems

COLONIZATION
Presence of multiplying microorganism with no overt host immunologic reaction

LOCAL INFECTION
Presence of inflammatory response and tissue injury due to the ability of the multiplying microorganism to invade viable surrounding tissues

SYSTEMIC INFECTION
The presence of the microorganisms in the blood stream causing systemic immune response

Exposed wound surfaces provides ideal culture medium for a wide varieties of microorganisms to contaminate and colonized. Multiplication of bacteria within a wound can reach a state of 'critical colonization' where the bacteria will invade viable tissues and leads to infection.

The abundance and diversity of bacteria in any wound depends on wound type, depth, location, the quality of the tissues, the level of tissue perfusion, and host immune response.

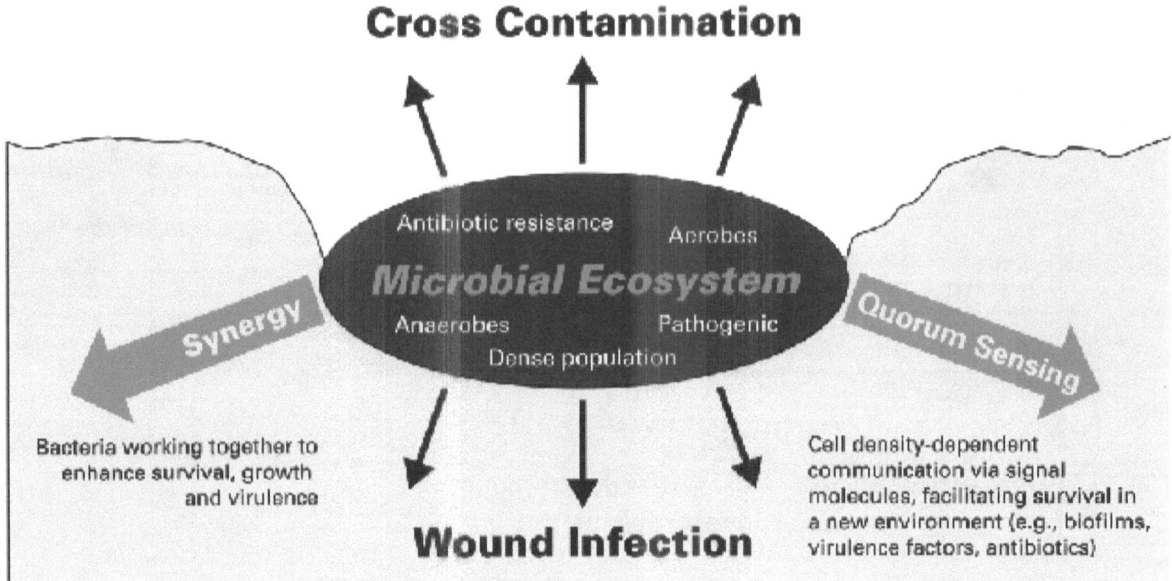

Figure 4-1 Wound microbial ecosystem

The microbial ecosystem in a wound is very dynamic and is usually polymicrobial. Some growing bacteria produce specific nutrients that promote the growth of certain fastidious pathogenic cohabiting bacteria while others consume the oxygen in the wound environment and induce tissue hypoxia thus leading to the growth of anaerobic bacteria.

This synergistic actions plus the use of quorum sensing between the bacteria leads to tissues invasion as well as promoting selection for resistant gene. The presence of multi-resistant gene in the wound leads to cross – contamination to other patients in the ward.

4-2. Common Pathogenic Bacteria Isolated from Different Types of Wound

Type of wound	Probable aerobic bacteria	Probable anaerobic bacteria
Surgical wound	*Staphylococcus aureus* Enterococcus sp *Pseudomonas aeruginosa* *Escherichia coli* Enterobacter sp *(depends on the site and type of surgery)*	contaminated wounds or dirty wounds may contain anaerobes especially those involving hollow viscous

SECTION A: BASIC WOUND PRINCIPLE | 20

Traumatic wound	Staphylococcus aureus Pseudomonas aeruginosa Escherichia coli Streptococcus pyogenes Klebsiella pneumoniae	Clostridium spp.
Bite wound (Polymicrobial)	Staphylococcus aureus Streptococcus spp Less common – Pasturella multocida/ Pasturella canis/ Capnocytophaga canimorsus/ B. Henselae / E. corrodens	Bacteroides spp Provotella spp Peptostreptococcus spp Clostridium perfringens
Diabetic foot ulcer (polymicrobial)	Staphylococcus aureus Streptococcua agalactiae (GBS) Pseudomonas aeruginosa Enterococcus spp Coliforms	Peptostreptococcus Bacteroides spp Provotella
Decubitus ulcer	Staphylococcus aureus Pseudomonas aeruginosa	Peptostreptococcus Bacteroides spp
HealthCare Associated Infection (HCAI) wound (formerly known as nosocomial infection)	Multi Resistant Staphylococcus aureus Extended Spectrum Beta Lactamases MRO: Acinetobacter spp Pseudomonas aeruginosa	

Type of Wound	Probable Aerobic Bacteria	Probable Anaerobic Bacteria
Burn wound	Pseudomonas aeruginosa/ Staphylococcus aureus/ Escherichia coli/ Klebsiella spp/ Enterococcus spp	Peptostreptococcus Bacteroides spp Propionibacterium acne

Wounds that is likely to contain anaerobic bacteria:

- Wounds that are in close proximity to the mucosal areas
- Wounds that are deep and contains devitalized tissues (Necrotizing fasciitis/ gas gangrene)
- Chronic non healing wounds with poor blood perfusion

4-3. Microbial Analysis of Wounds

Analysis of wound microbiology i.e. culture & sensitivity (C&S) **should not** be done routinely. Four situations where sampling is recommended:

i. Wounds that have clinical signs and symptoms of infection

Triggers For Suspecting Wound Infection in Wounds	
1. New or increase swelling	5. Purulent discharge or increase in the level of exudates
2. Local warmth	6. Discoloration of surrounding skin
3. Erythema or further extension of erythema	7. Wound breakdown / dehiscence
4. New or increasing pain	8. Lymphangitis
	9. Fever

ii. Extensive burn wound (> 20%)
iii. Suspicious wound with implant, vascular graft or skin graft rejection
iv. Chronic non-healing wounds

4-4. Specimen Collection

1. *Wound swabbing*
   - Test request: Wound swab for C&S
   - Suitable for superficial wounds
   - Requirements:

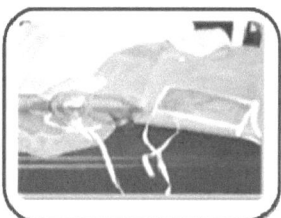 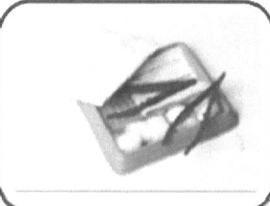 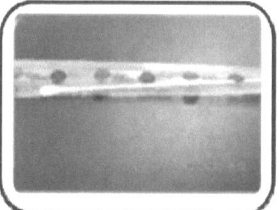 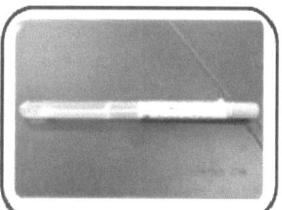

1. Appropriate PPE as per Infection Control Guidelines
2. Dressing pack
3. Sterile cotton tipped swab
4. Transport medium

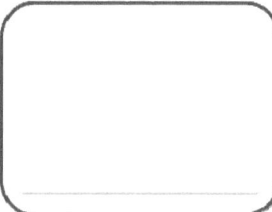 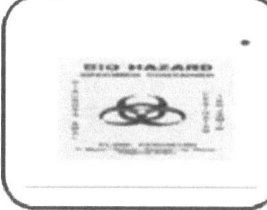 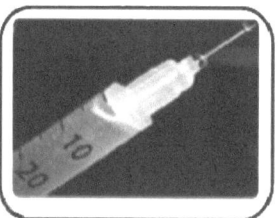

5. PER PATH 301 form
6. Biohazard plastic container
7. Syringe and needle for irrigation

Procedure for Wound Swab C&S
1. Prepare the required equipments as above
2. Perform hand hygiene and wear PPE
3. Clean the wound using sterile water or saline. Irrigate the wound surface using syringe and needle to flush out contaminating and colonizing bacteria
4. Moist the sterile swab (if the wound surface is dry) with normal saline
5. Use a zigzag motion whilst simultaneously rotating the swab stick between the fingers
6. Sample the whole wound surface
7. Place the specimen straight into the transport medium and label the container
▪ Complete the request form (PER PATH 301). Clinical information should be provided (e.g., type and site of wound, associated malodor, signs of infection, antibiotic therapy) in order to ensure that meaningful results can be provided in as short a time as possible
8. Place the specimen and request form into the Biohazard bag and send straight to the laboratory
9. Store wound swabs at room temperature

2. *Tissue sampling*
   - Test request : Tissue for C&S and gram stain
   - Should be performed aseptically after initial debridement and cleansing (with sterile saline or distilled water) of the wound

Procedure for Tissue Sampling	
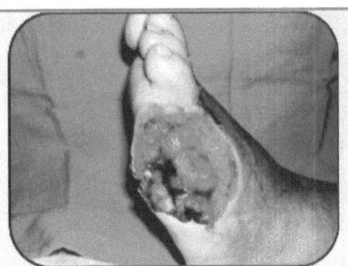	Obtain tissue sample from the deep part of the wound or base of the lesion/wound/ulcer and placed into a sterile screw capped container with few drops of saline to keep it moist

3. *Fluid sampling*
   - Test request: Fluids for C&S and gram stain
   - Suitable for wound with cavity, sinus or pockets. Should be done aseptically after cleansing (with sterile saline or distilled water)

Procedure for Fluid Sampling	
1. Place about 5 ml of aspirate in a sterile screw capped bottle 2. If the pus is very little, use a sterile swab to collect a sample from the cavity or sinus and immerse the swab in the transport medium 3. Send the specimen immediately to the lab 4. Sample should be taken from deep cavity or sinus	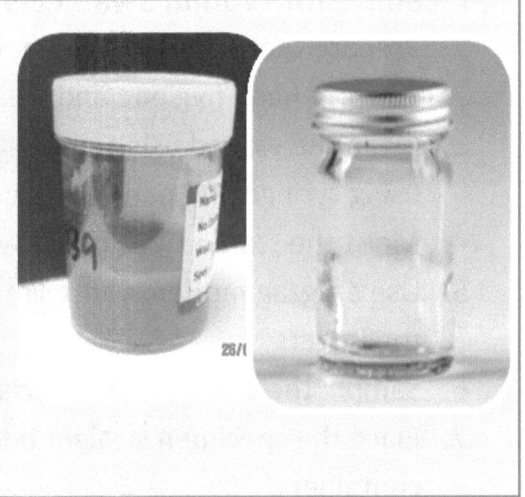

4. *Anaerobic Culture Collection*
   - Test request: Tissues or fluids for C&S and gram stain
   - Should be done aseptically
   - Samples must be either aspirates or tissues only. **Swabs are not suitable for anaerobic culture**
   - Small tissue sample should be placed in an aerobic transport media or Robertson cooked meat medium.
   - Larger tissue sample (≥ 1 cm) can be placed in a screw capped bottle.
   - The bigger the tissue, the higher is the yield for anaerobic culture

Storage and Transportation of Wound Specimens	
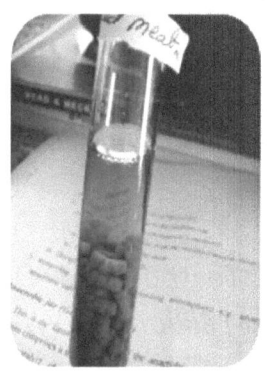	1. Specimens should be sent immediately to the laboratory for processing 2. In hospitals where the laboratory does not accept specimens after office hours or over the weekends, the specimen should be kept at room temperature and sent immediately on the next working day.

4-5. Antibiotic Treatment

- Antibiotics should only be given when there is evidence of wound infection
- Should follow the antibiotic guideline
- Empirical treatment should cover the possible organisms as stated in the table 4-2 above or follow the local antimicrobial pattern and should be changed according to the C&S results

Point to Remember:

- Surface swab has the lowest clinical value
- Sample should be taken when indicated
- Correct sampling technique is pertinent for optimal yield
- Antibiotic treatment only initiated when indicated and must follow guideline

Reference

1. Bowler P. G, Duerden B. I & Armstrong D. G. Wound Microbiology and Associated. Approaches to Wound Management. Clin. Microbiol. Rev, Vol 14, No 2, pp 244 – 269

2. Jousimies – Somer H, et al. Anaerobic Bacteriology Manual, 2002, 6th Ed. Helsinki: Star Publishing Company.

3. Winn WC, et al. Koneman's Color Atlas and Textbook of Diagnostic Microbiology, 2006, 6TH Ed. Baltimore: Lippincott Milliams & Wilkins

4. Wound Care Guidelines, Bolton Primary Care Nhs Trust & Bolton Hospitals Nhs Trust. www.bolton.nhs.uk/Library/policies/Nurswc001.pdf

CHAPTER 5: Nutrition in Wound Care

Pn Harizah Mohd Yaacob / Pn Mageswary Lapshmanan/ Pn Nurul Huda Ibrahim

Learning Objectives:

1. To understand the importance of nutrition in wound healing
2. To identify patients with malnutrition and at risk for malnutrition
3. To be able to prescribe basic nutrition care

5-1. Introduction

Provision of nutritional care is proven to accelerate wound healing. Appropriate nutritional screening and early nutrition intervention is a fundamental **component** of wound management. Poor nutrition before or during the recovery process may delay healing and impair wound strength, making the wound more prone to breakdown.

Healthcare professionals can help reduce the morbidity, mortality and cost associated with chronic wounds by combining knowledge of the wound healing process with good nutrition support practices.

5-2. Nutrition Screening

Nutrition Screening should be done early to identify patients with malnutrition or at risk for malnutrition using Malnutrition Universal Screening Tool (MUST) as in Figure 5-1.

Patients who are at risk for malnutrition include:

- Patients with chronic wound
- Patients with non-healing wound
- Patients with infected wound
- Uncontrolled DM patients with ulcer
- Underweight patients
- Bed bound patients
- Burn patients

Patients with co-morbidities such as uncontrolled diabetes mellitus, dyslipidemia, cancer, kidney diseases and hypertension are recommended to consult or refer a dietitian.

MALNUTRITION UNIVERSAL SCREENING TOOL (MUST)

Step 1 — BMI score

BMI kg/m²	Score
>20 (>30 Obese)	= 0
18.5-20	= 1
<18.5	= 2

If unable to obtain height and weight, see reverse for alternative measurements and use of subjective criteria

Step 2 — Weight loss score

Unplanned weight loss in past 3-6 months

%	Score
<5	= 0
5-10	= 1
>10	= 2

Step 3 — Acute disease effect score

If patient is acutely ill **and** there has been or is likely to be no nutritional intake for >5 days
Score 2

Acute disease effect is unlikely to apply outside hospital. See 'MUST' Explanatory Booklet for further information

Step 4 — Overall risk of malnutrition

Add Scores together to calculate overall risk of malnutrition
Score 0 Low Risk   Score 1 Medium Risk   Score 2 or more High Risk

Step 5 — Management guidelines

0 Low Risk — Routine clinical care
- Repeat screening
  Hospital – weekly
  Care Homes – monthly
  Community – annually for special groups e.g. those >75 yrs

1 Medium Risk — Observe
- Document dietary intake for 3 days
- If adequate – little concern and repeat screening
  • Hospital – weekly
  • Care Home – at least monthly
  • Community – at least every 2-3 months
- If inadequate – clinical concern – follow local policy, set goals, improve and increase overall nutritional intake, monitor and review care plan regularly

2 or more High Risk — Treat*
- Refer to dietitian, Nutritional Support Team or implement local policy
- Set goals, improve and increase overall nutritional intake
- Monitor and review care plan
  Hospital – weekly
  Care Home – monthly
  Community – monthly

* Unless detrimental or no benefit is expected from nutritional support e.g. imminent death.

All risk categories:
- Treat underlying condition and provide help and advice on food choices, eating and drinking when necessary.
- Record malnutrition risk category.
- Record need for special diets and follow local policy.

Obesity:
- Record presence of obesity. For those with underlying conditions, these are generally controlled before the treatment of obesity.

Re-assess subjects identified at risk as they move through care settings

*Adopted from Malnutrition Advisory Group (MAG), a standing committee of BAPEN, August 2011

Figure 5.1 Malnutrition universal screening tool (MUST)

5-3. Nutrition Management

Optimal wound healing requires adequate nutrition as well as involvement of wound management team, effective communication and compliance to standard protocol.

Wound healing is a complex process – in simple terms, it is the process of replacing injured tissue with new tissue, which demands an increased consumption of energy and particular nutrients. A wound causes a number of changes in the body that can affect the healing process, including changes in energy, protein, carbohydrate, fat, vitamin and mineral metabolism. The body experiences catabolic phase with an increased metabolic rate, loss of total body water, and increased collagen and cellular turnover.

If the catabolic phase is prolonged and the body is not provided with adequate nutrient supplies, the body can enter a protein energy malnutrition (PEM) state. The severity of the wound and the preexisting nutritional status of the individual can lead to prolonged catabolism.

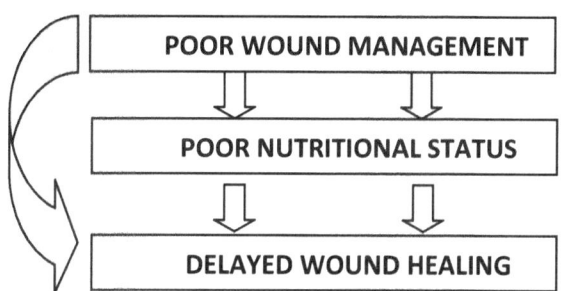

PEM causes the body to break down protein for energy, reducing the supply of amino acids needed to maintain body proteins and healing, and causing loss of lean body mass delayed wound healing. **When a patient loses more lean body mass (LBM), wound healing is more likely to be delayed. With a 20% or greater loss of LBM, wounds compete with muscles for nutrients. If LBM loss reaches 30% or more, the body will often prioritise the rebuilding of body over wound healing with protein available.**

Thus, appropriate and timely nutrition support is essential to attenuate hypermetabolisme and hypercatabolisme and help wound healing.

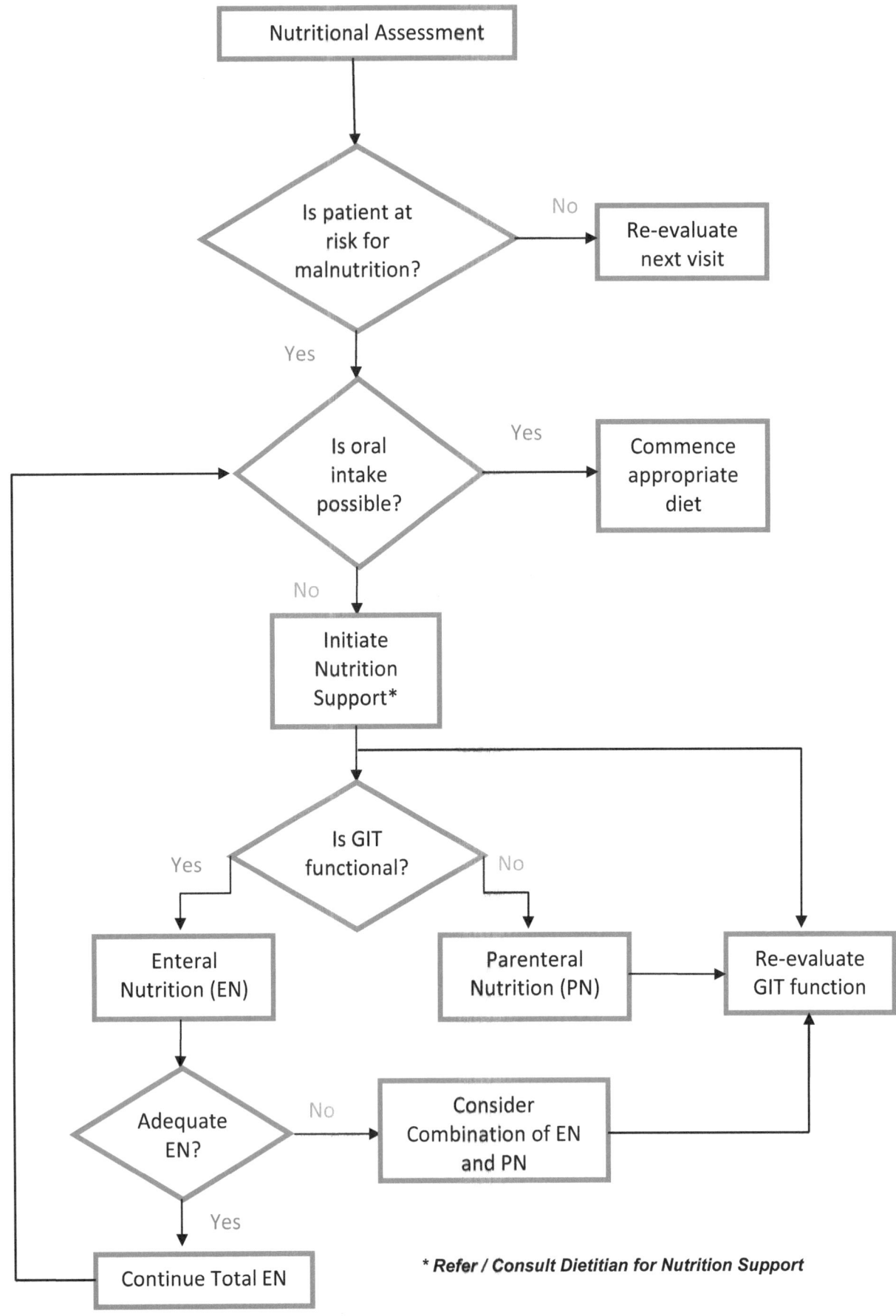

Figure 5.2 Algorithm for nutrition management

5-4. Nutrition Prescription

1. Nutrient Recommendation

Provision of some specific nutrients has been shown to promote wound healing. Age-appropriate protein and energy needs should be provided. Nutritional supplements with enteral or parenteral support should be considered if target needs are not achieved. Suspected or confirmed micronutrient deficiency should be treated early with provision of 100% RNI (Recommended Nutrient Intake) of micronutrients.

Table 5.1 Recommended intake for wound healing

Nutrient	Recommended Intake
Energy	<ul><li>Underweight : 35 – 45 kcal/kg/day</li><li>Normal : 30 – 35 kcal/kg/day</li><li>Overweight : 25 – 30 kcal/kg/day</li><li>Burn : 40 kcal/kg/day</li><li>Trauma : 35 – 45 kcal/kg/day</li></ul>
Carbohydrate	<ul><li>50 – 60% of Energy</li><li>DM: Encourage high fibre complex CHO e.g. wholegrain bread, capati, brown rice according to recommended serving sizes</li></ul>
Fat	<ul><li>30 – 35% of Energy</li><li>Adult : 0.8 – 1.5 g/kg/day</li><li>Dyslipidemia : Limit high saturated fat and fried food</li></ul>
Protein	<ul><li>Chronic wound : 1.25 – 1.5 g/kg/day</li><li>Severely catabolic with more than one wound or Pressure Ulcers Stage III & IV : 1.5 – 2.0 g/kg/day</li><li>Vegetarian : consume enough protein from milk, lentils, legumes and beans</li></ul>
Pharmaconutrients	<ul><li>Omega-3 fatty acid</li><li>Linoleic acid</li><li>L-Glutamine 0.2 – 0.5 g/kg/day</li><li>Arginine 30 – 60 g/day</li></ul>
Vitamin A	<ul><li>Malnourished patient : 1000 IU</li><li>Severe burn, poor nutrient store, GI dysfunction, radiation therapy : 10,000 – 25,000 IU</li><li>At least 1 serving per day of dark, green &leafy vegetables, orange or yellow vegetables, orange fruit, liver and fortified dairy products</li></ul>

Vitamin B Complex	- B1 (Thiamine) : 10 mg/day - B2 (Riboflavine) : 10 mg/day - B3 (Niacin) : 200 mg/day - B5 (Pantothenic acid) : 100 mg/day - B6 (Pyridoxine) : 20 mg/day - B7 (Biotin) : 5 mg/day - B9 (Folic acid) : 2 mg/day - B12 (Cobalamine) : 20 µg/day

Vitamin C	- Small wound eg. Pressure ulcers /elective small to moderate surgery:
	    ➤ 0.5 – 1 g daily in 2 divided dosage
	- Larger injury eg: large BSA burn & Multiple trauma:
	    ➤ 1 – 2 g/day
	- At least 1 serving per day of citrus fruits, guava, tomato, pepper, potatoes, spinach and cruciferous (broccoli, cabbage, cauliflower)

Vitamin E	Not to exceed 670mg/day
Vitamin K	5-10mg (orally or IM 1-3 times weekly in high risk patients)
Zinc	- 40 mg/day for 10 days - Red meats, seafood and fortified cereals
Selenium	100 µg/day
Manganese	25 – 50 mg/day
Copper	2 – 3 mg/day

Table 5.2 Recommended food intake for wound healing

Food Group	1 Serving Size	Daily Serving (Normal Recommendation)	Daily Serving (Wound Healing Recommendation)
Rice, noodle, bread, cereals, cereal products and tubers	1 cup @ 2 scoops rice / noodles / cereals 2 slices bread 1 capati / thosai	4 – 8 servings	4 – 8 servings
Vegetables	½ cup @ 2 table spoons leafy (spinach, kangkung) or starchy (carrots, potato)	2 – 3 servings	4 servings
Fruits	1 slice papaya/ pineapple /honeydew / watermelon 1 whole apple/ orange	2 servings	3 servings
Fish, poultry, meat and legume	1 fish (eg. kembung, selar) 1 drumstick 2 eggs 2 table spoons beef 1 cup @ 2 scoops cooked dhall 2 tauhu/ tempeh	2 – 3 servings	3 – 4 servings
Milk and milk products	1 cup milk 1 slice of cheese ¾ cup yogurt	1 – 3 servings	1 – 3 servings
Fats, oil, sugar and salt	1 tsp oil 1 tsp sugar 1 tsp salt	Eat less	Eat less

If patient not eating well;

1. Suggest five to six small meals a day. Encourage smaller meals and snacks between meals to get enough nutrition. Make nutritious snacks like mixed porridge, milk, hot chocolate, ice-cream, yogurt, fruits, sandwiches, milkshake, oats with milk, omelettes, *'roti telur'*, cream mushroom soup,

fruit or fruit juices, 'cekodok', pancakes, banana fritters, popcorn and corn in cup. Use foods that are "high nutrient-dense" as below:

"Low nutrient-dense" foods	"High nutrient-dense" foods
Clear soup (air rebusan)	Chicken / beef vegetable soup
Plain jelly	Jelly with milk / fruits
Carbonated beverages	Milk, milkshakes
Popsicles	Ice cream floats, smoothie, , ice cream
Plain bread / biscuits / pancake	Bread / biscuits / pancake with peanut butter / egg / tuna / sardine
Plain porridge	Chicken porridge, Fish porridge

2. Suggest variety of foods if patient experience taste changes to find out what works for the patient. Cold foods and foods with little odor work best. Add spices (e.g. lemongrass, pandan leaves, lime, mint leaves, herbs) in meat, chicken, fish preparations. Take lemon/ orange/ mint flavoured food or drinks to reduce the metallic or bitter taste.

3. Use an oral nutritional supplement if nothing else works. These are available at grocery stores, drug stores, and hypermarkets. Adding milk, cocoa powder, coffee or ice cream may make the supplement tastier.

4. Take a multivitamin if unable to meet the recommended intake (Refer Appendix 1).

Diabetes Mellitus or Hypertensive

Continue to monitor blood sugar levels closely. Having good control of blood sugar levels will help with wound healing and may prevent infection. Consult a doctor and a dietitian to help control blood sugar through diet and medication.

Consult and refer to a dietitian if patient's appetite remains poor, patient's wound is not healing well, and/or patient is losing weight.

5.5 Food Myth and Truth

MYTH	TRUTH
Haruan fish and 'ikan linang' are strongly recommended after surgery for wound healing	Protein is essential for wound healing. Haruan fish and 'ikan linang / belut' are good source of protein similar to any other fish. Consume adequate protein from all type of fish, chicken, meat, lentils and beans to promote wound healing. Do not restrict to haruan fish or 'ikan linang' only.
Eggs will induce itchiness, pus and can cause wound breakdown.	Eggs are considered a complete protein source and rich in vitamins and minerals. There is no evidence that consumption of eggs and egg products are related to itchiness, pus and can cause wound breakdown. Only avoid eggs if you are allergic to it.
Female chicken meat should not be consumed after surgery.	Chicken meat is a good source of protein and there is no evidence of contraindication after surgery.
Application of gamat oil on wound and drinking gamat essence can help wound healing.	There is no strong research and evidence for the claim. Usually, any type of essence like essence of chicken, essence of haruan fish and gamat are high in salt and not advisable for regular consumption.

> **Point to Remember:**
>
> - Nutrition is essential for the wound-healing process
>
> - The most basic essential nutrients needed for wound healing are calories, protein, vitamins A and C, iron and zinc.
>
> - The use of a nutritional screening tool highlights those at risk of nutritional deficiency
>
> - Regular ongoing monitoring is necessary to evaluate the outcome of nutrition intervention and manage feeding barriers effectively

Reference

1. Molner JA. Nutrition and wound healing. CRC Press UK 2007.

2. Abdul Rahman MJ, Mohd Fuad M, Prusat K, Khalit S. Fatty acid compositions in mucus and roe of Haruan, Channa Striatus, for wound healing. General Pharmacology: The Vascular System 1998; 30(4): 561 – 563.

3. Collins C. Nutrition and wound care. Clinical Nutrition Highlight 2006; 2(3): 1 – 2.

4. T Wild et al. Basics in nutrition and wound healing review article. Nutrition 2010; 26(9): 862 – 966.

5. Malaysian Dietary Guidelines. Ministry of Health Malaysia 2010.

Chapter 6: Principles of Wound Closure

Dr. Normala Hj. Basiron

6-1. Introduction

The goal of treating any type of wound is to create an optimal wound healing environment by producing a well vascularised, stable wound bed that is conducive to normal and timely healing. In addition, the ultimate aims of wound closure include:
- Safety i.e. immediate success of wound closure and ensure preservation of life or limb
- Restoration of form with optimal aesthetic outcome
- Preservation of function

6-2. Principles of wound closure

1. Perform general and local wound assessment. (refer to Chapter 3 – Wound assessment and documentation)
2. Perform wound or defect analysis by assessing:
    - Location - whether near or exposing the vital organs or structures
    - Size – small or large
    - Physical components involvement – type of soft tissues like muscle, tendon and nerve or bone
3. Multidisciplinary approach to treat the underlying causes or problems of unstable wound hence managing the patient in the holistic manner.
4. Wound closure by replacing tissue defect "like with like" tissue (appropriate tissue match) whenever possible.
5. Choose appropriate technique of wound closure ensuring safety, preservation of function and aesthetically pleasing.

6-3. Types of wounds in perspective of wound closure

1. Simple wounds

Wounds that are readily managed by local wound care with subsequent contraction (healing by secondary intension), primary closure, split thickness skin graft (SSG), or local tissue/ flap rearrangement.

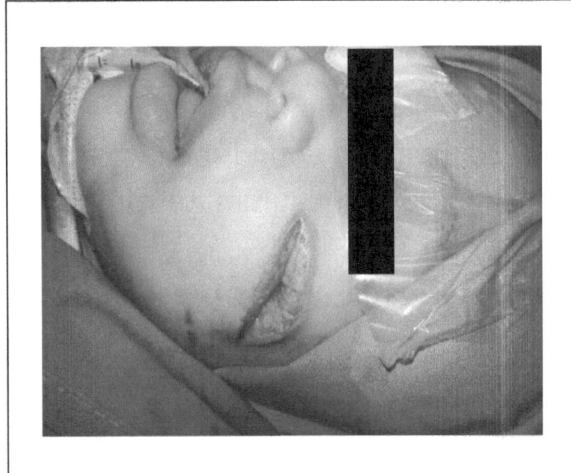

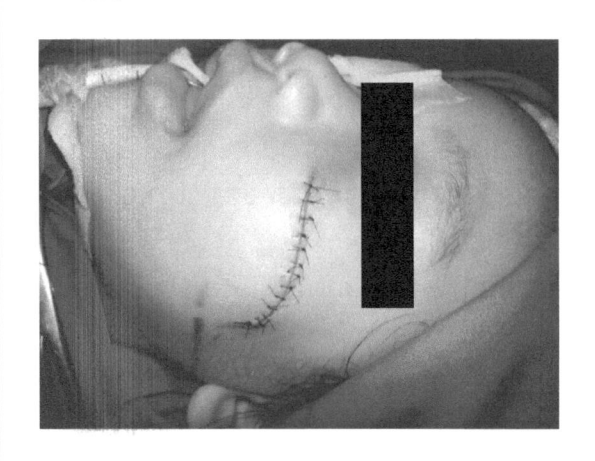

Figure 6.1 Example of simple wound with primary closure

2. Complex wounds

Wounds that have excessive depth or size, in an unfavorable location, limb or life threatening conditions that usually require a distant pedicled tissue flap transposition or by microsurgery tissue flap transplantation (free flap) for closure.

Figure 6.2 (a) Example of complex wound after cancer extirpation**

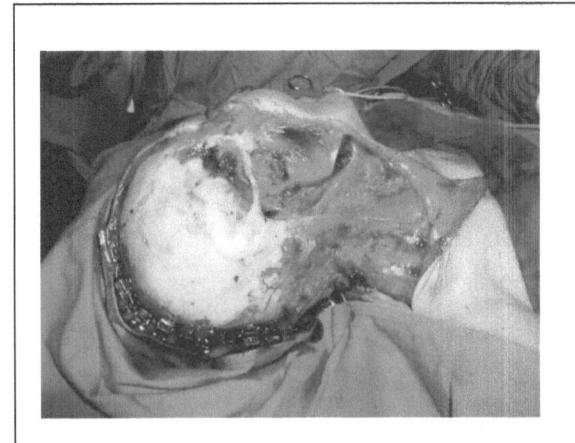

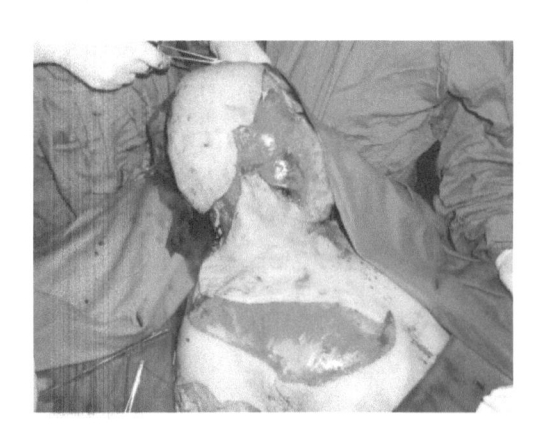

Figure 6.2 (b) Pedicled flap raised from chestwall and neck to cover the lower portion of wound. Transverse Rectus Abdominis Myocutaneous free flap to cover the upper portion of the wound.

SECTION A: BASIC WOUND PRINCIPLE | 38

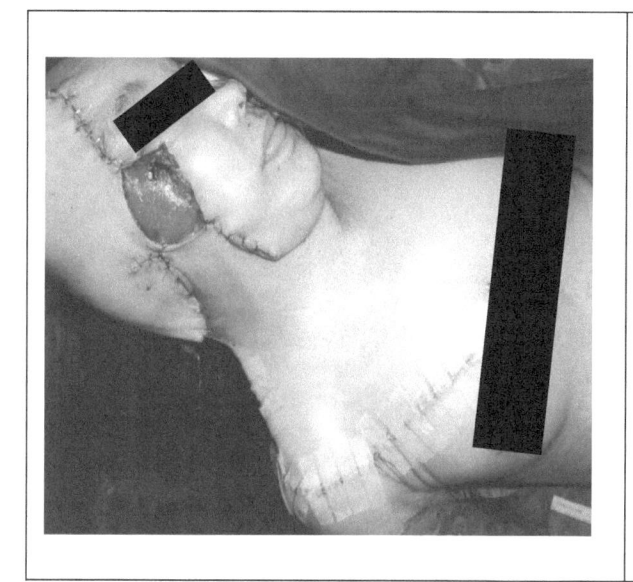

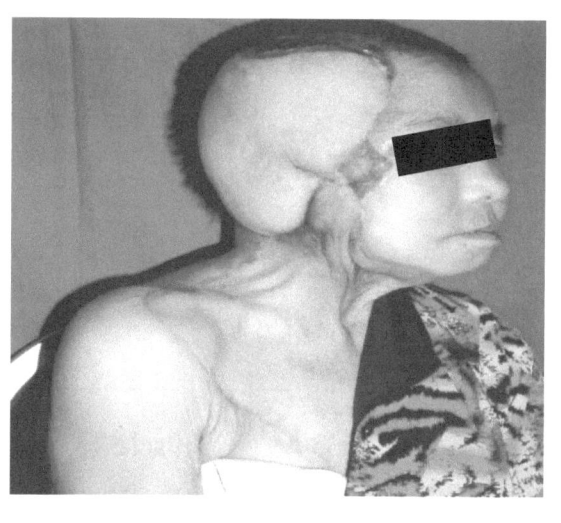

* **extirpation** - *removing solid matter from a part of the body*

Figure 6.2(c) Complex wound closed with combination of SSG, local pedicled flap and free flap

Figure 6.2(d) Three months post surgery

3. **Unstable wounds**

   Wound recurrence after a simple or complex wound closure technique or due to other related causes of wounds.

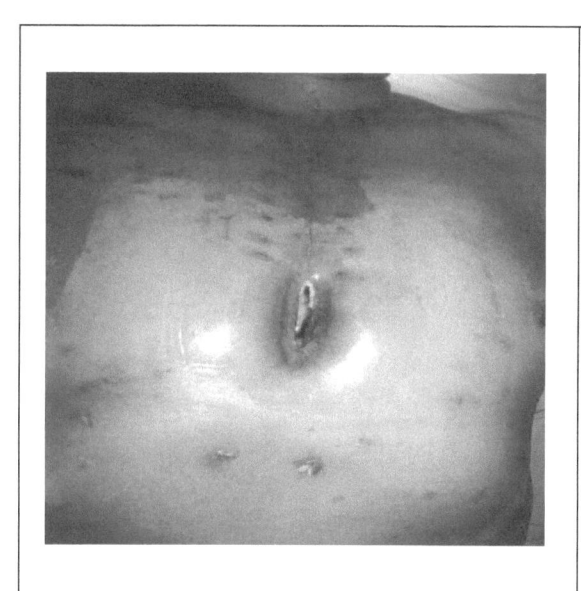

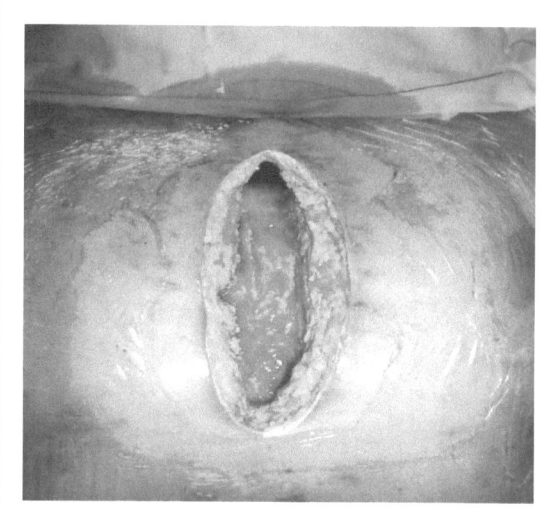

Figure 6.3(a) Example of wound breakdown and mediastinitis after sternotomy

Figure 6.3(b) After wound debridement

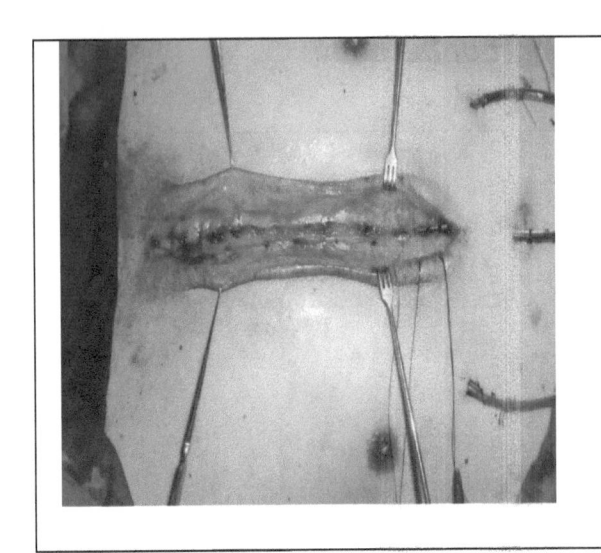

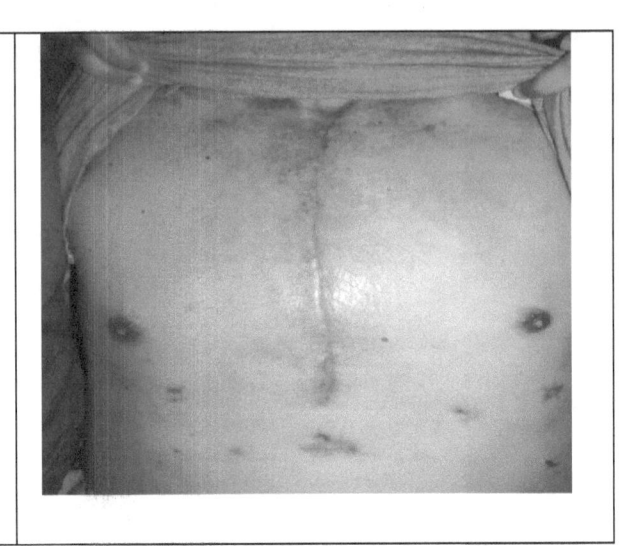

Figure 6.3 (c) After muscle flap repair

Figure 6.3 (d) After primary closure

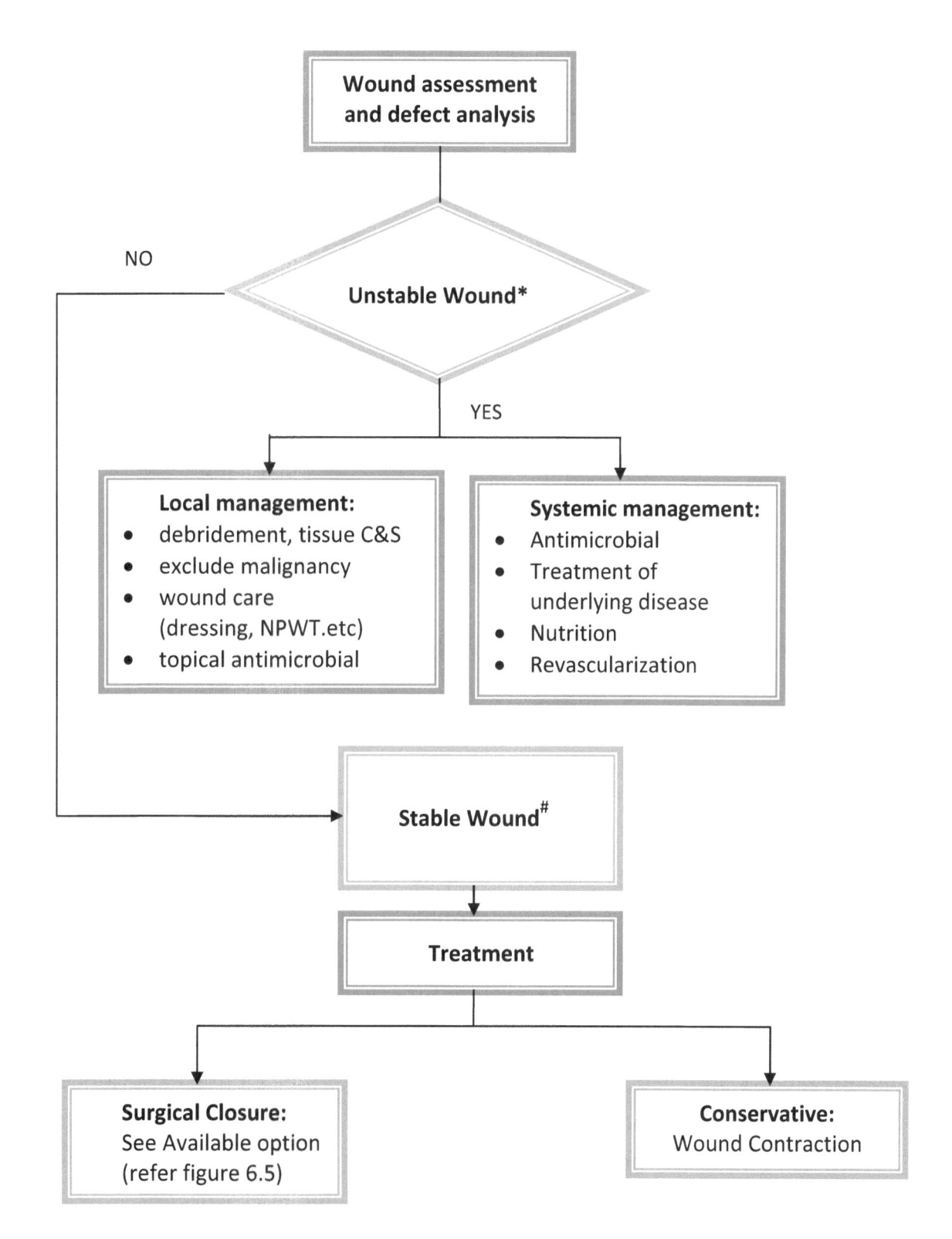

6-4. Principles in Wound Closure & Reconstruction Planning

```
          Wound assessment
          and defect analysis
                   │
                   ▼
NO ◄────────  Unstable Wound*
                   │ YES
         ┌─────────┴─────────┐
         ▼                   ▼
  Local management:    Systemic management:
  • debridement,       • Antimicrobial
    tissue C&S         • Treatment of
  • exclude malignancy   underlying disease
  • wound care         • Nutrition
    (dressing,         • Revascularization
    NPWT.etc)
  • topical antimicrobial

                ▼
          Stable Wound#
                │
                ▼
           Treatment
         ┌──────┴──────┐
         ▼             ▼
  Surgical Closure:  Conservative:
  See Available      Wound Contraction
  option
  (refer figure 6.5)
```

Figure 6.4 Algorithm converting an unstable wound to a stable wound prior to the treatment

Wound assessment method – refer T.I.M.E. principle
* Unstable wound- wound not ready for closure
 # Stable wound- wound ready for closure

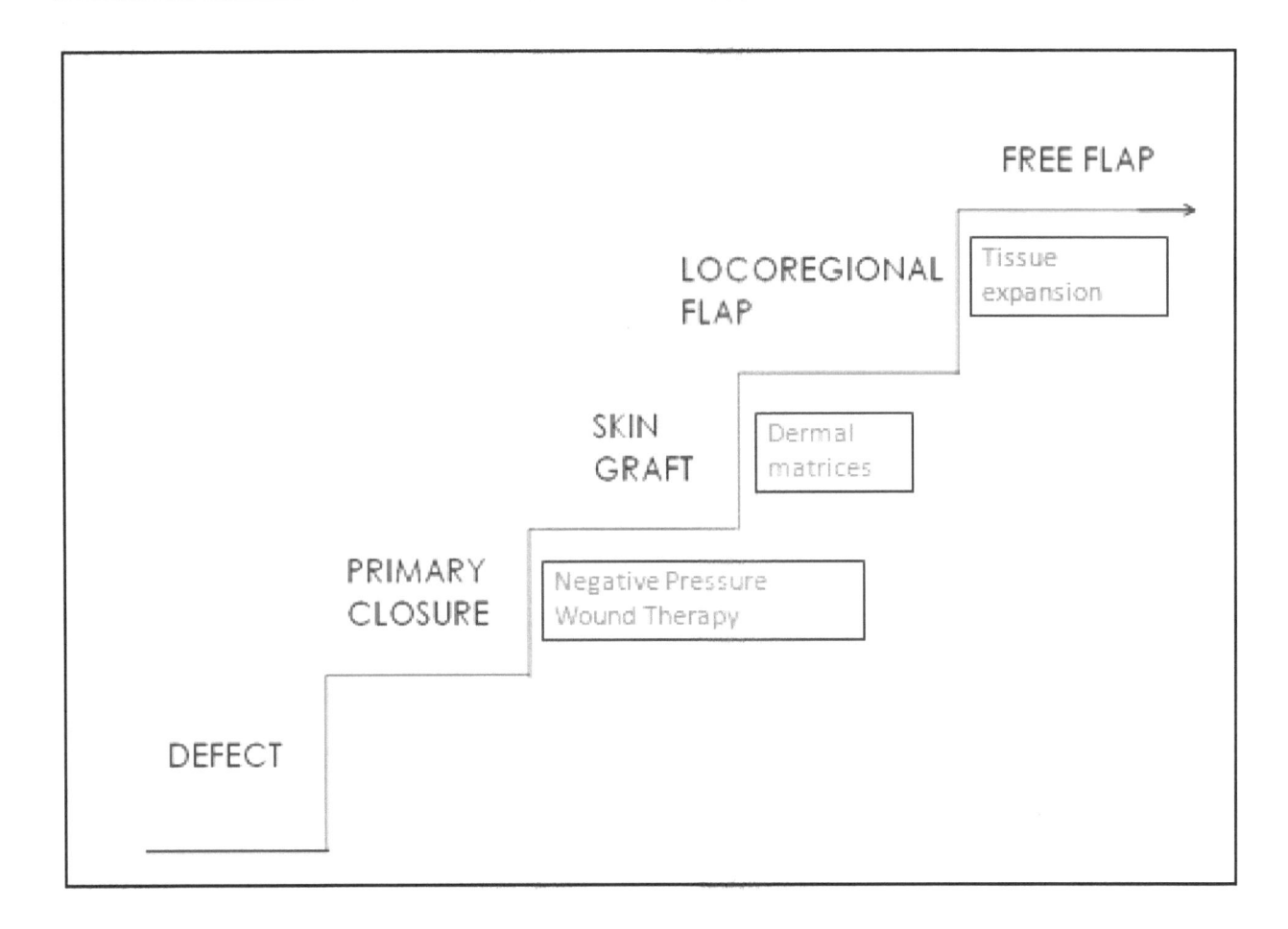

6-5. Options for Wound Closure and Reconstruction

Figure 6.5 Reconstructive Ladder

The reconstructive ladder provides a systematic approach to wound closure emphasizing selection of simple to complex techniques based on local wound requirements and complexity. Whenever it is indicated, closure of wound must not only safe and preserve form but also restore function. Nevertheless, selection of the wound closure techniques still needs to consider individual patient factors and also factors involving surgeons' judgments, experience and familiarity with the techniques and availability of services for advanced wound closure technique i.e. negative pressure wound therapy, dermal matrices or skin substitute like collagen, tissue expansion and flap microsurgery.

Table 6.1 Example of type of wound and its closure

Type Of Wound	Type Of Wound Closure
Simple wound	Wound contraction
Post trauma simple wound	Primary closure after bone fixation

Post trauma large simple wound	Negative pressure wound Therapy (refer chapter on NPWT)
Large simple wound post degloving injury after wound bed preparation showing healthy granulation tissue	Split thickness skin graft (SSG) closure of the wound

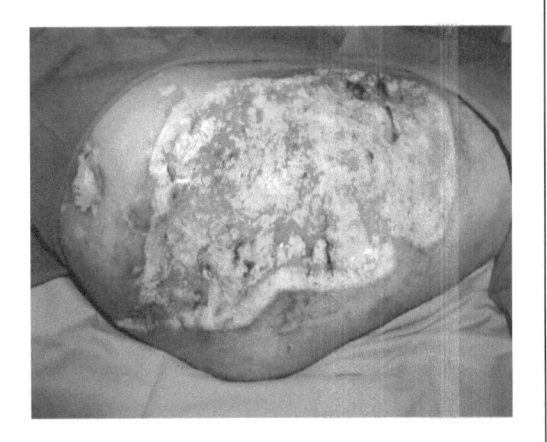

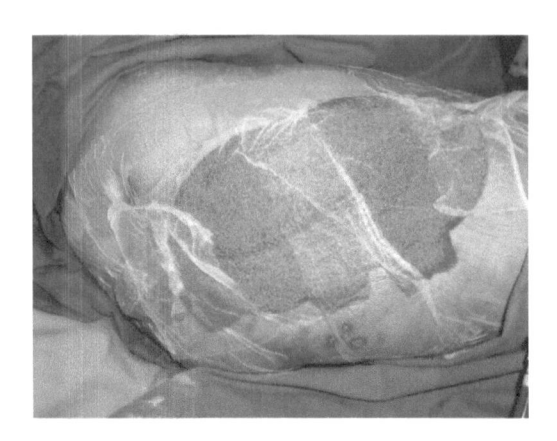

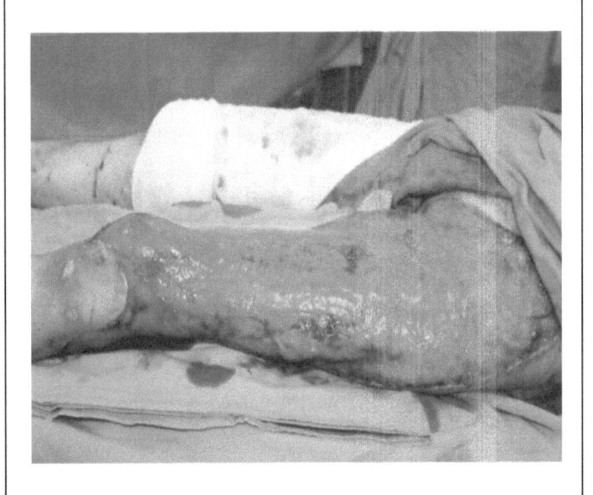

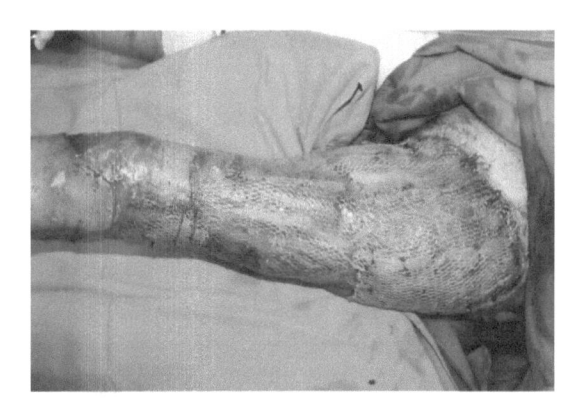

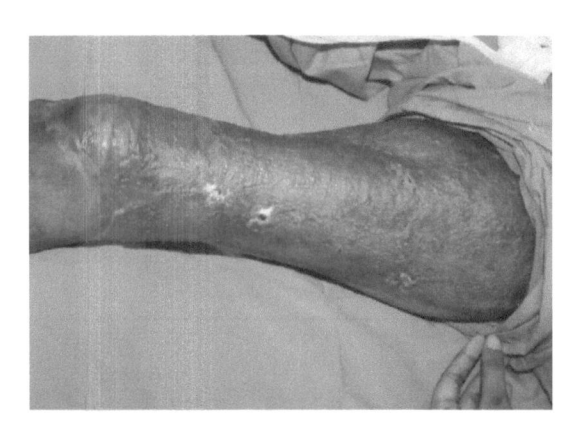

Almost 100% SSG has taken up and wound has healed nicely.

SECTION A: BASIC WOUND PRINCIPLE

Unstable wound post renal transplant surgery exposing viable and functioning transplanted kidney

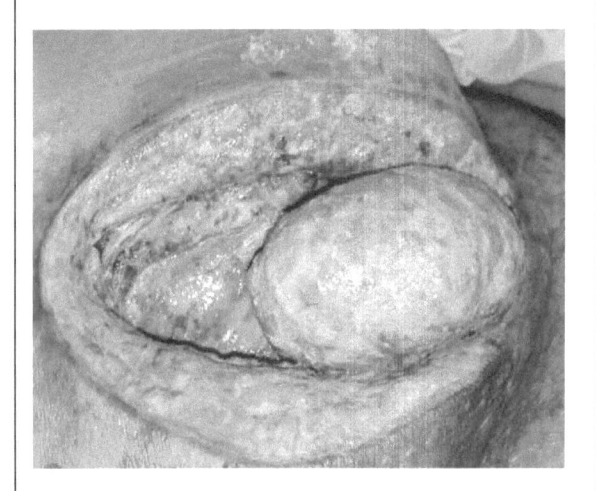

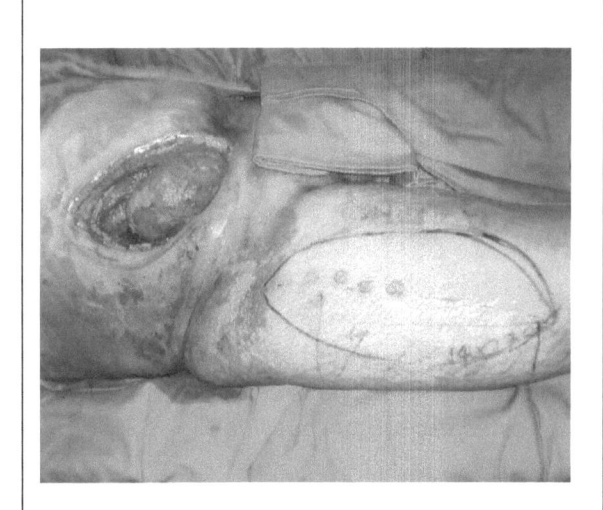

After debridement and wound bed preparation the wound is ready for closure.

Locoregional flap (pedicled flap) closure using anterolateral thigh fasciocutaneous flap

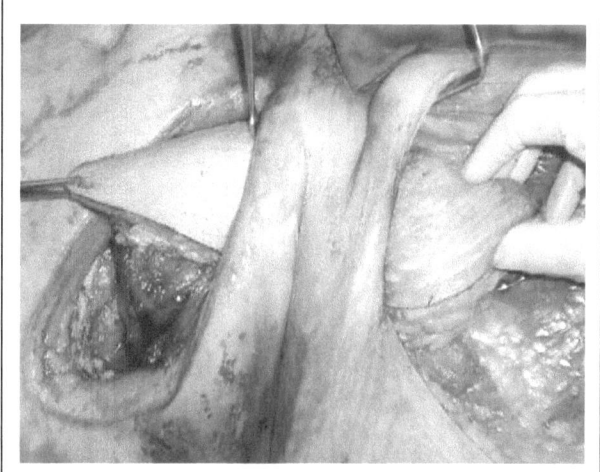

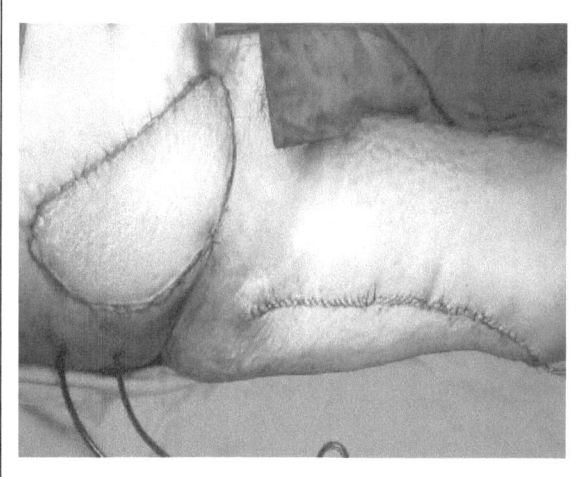

After inserting the flap to cover the kidney, the donor site wound in the thigh is closed primarily

Unstable wound post compound fracture right tibia/ fibula complicated with osteomyelitis

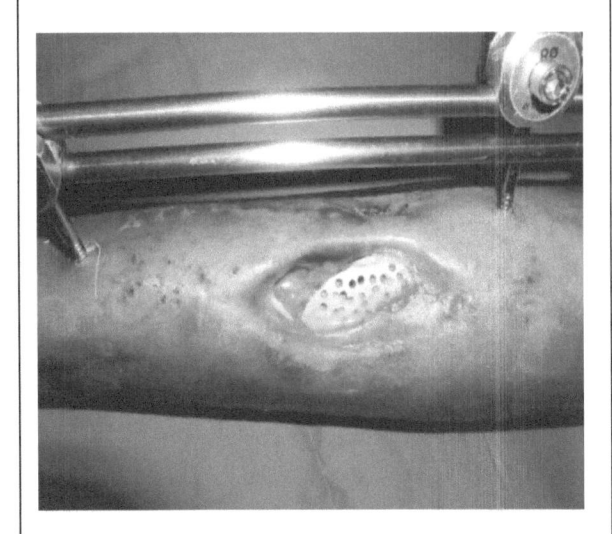

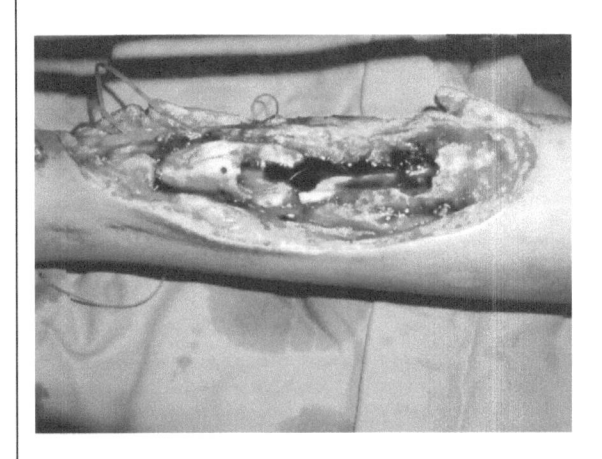

Wound after debridement and removal of osteomyelitic bone leaving a complex wound exposing a significant bone gap is ready for closure

Wound closure with free tissue/ flap transfer

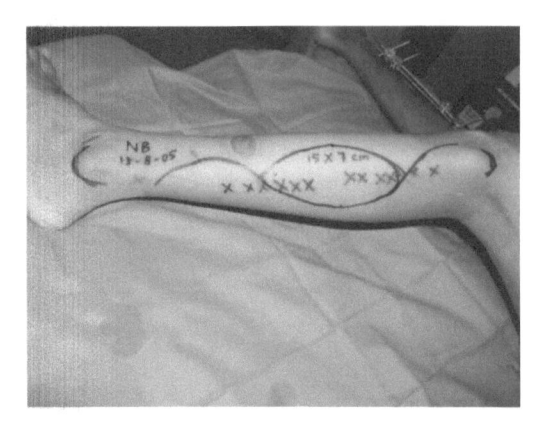

Fibula osteofasciocutaneous flap harvested from left lower limb

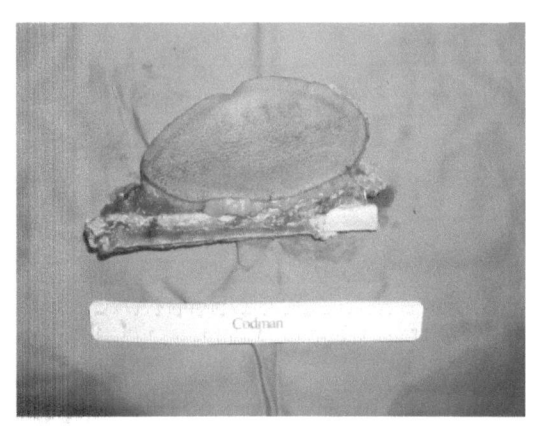

Bone gap and soft tissue defect reconstructed with free osteofasciocutaneous flap

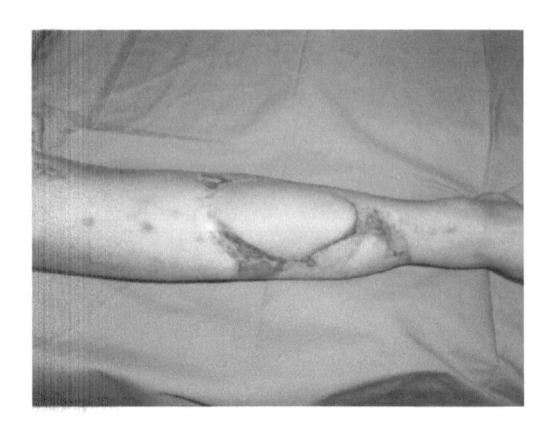

One year after surgery

SECTION A: BASIC WOUND PRINCIPLE | 46

6-6. How Does Flap Differ from Graft?

Flap	Graft
Definition	
Tissue that is mobilized on the basis of its vascular anatomy.	Transfer of tissue without its own blood supply (skin, bone, nerve or vein).
e.g. cutaneous, fasciocutaneous, osteofasciocutaneous, myocutaneous, muscle flap, etc.)	Survival of graft depends entirely on the blood supply from the recipient site.
Type	

1. **Pedicled flap/ locoregional flap**

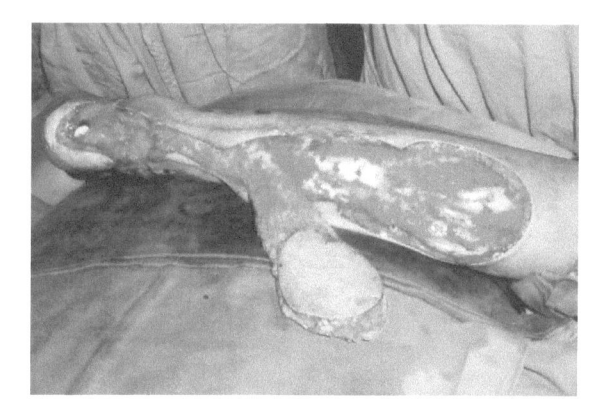

   Tissue transferred while still attached to its original blood supply.

2. **Free flap**

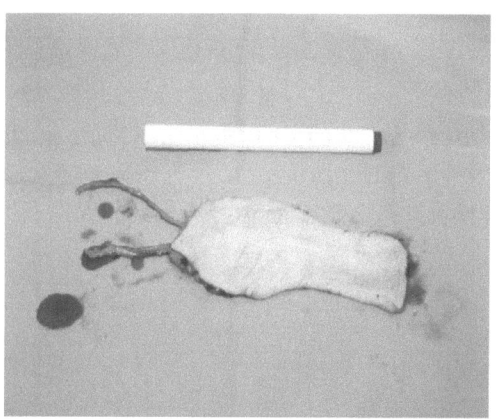

   Tissue transferred with physically detached from its native blood supply and then reattached to vessels at the recipient site by microsurgical anastomosis.

1. **Split thickness skin graft (SSG)**

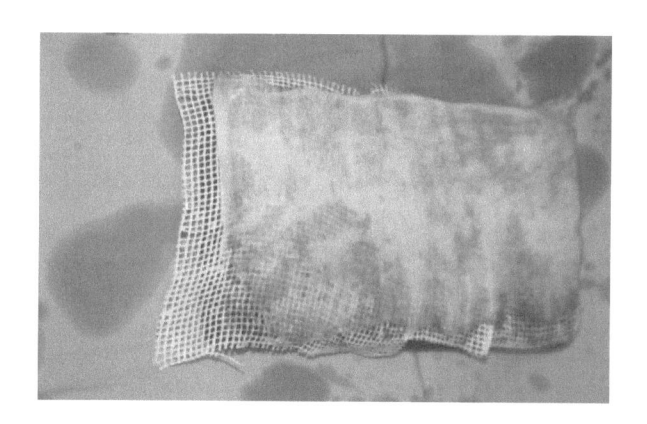

   Contains varying thickness of dermis

2. **Full thickness skin graft (FTG)**

   Contains the entire dermis

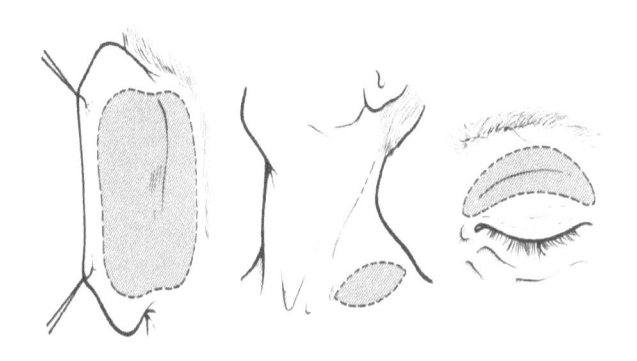

SECTION A: BASIC WOUND PRINCIPLE | 47

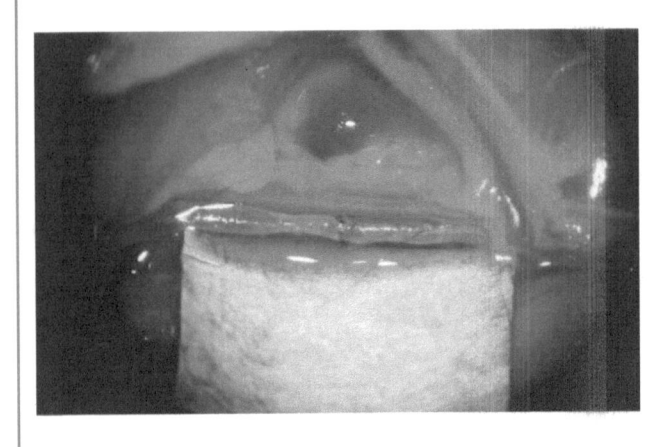

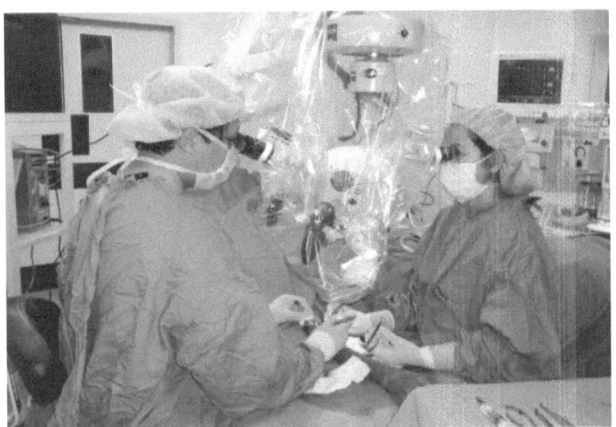

Blood vessels anastomosis under the microscope magnification

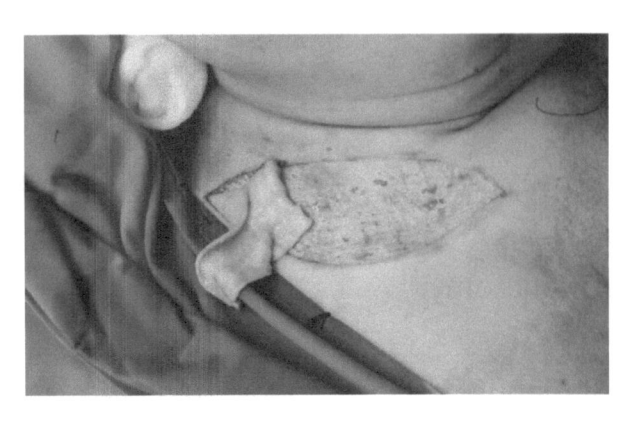

FTG harvested from supraclavicular skin for left cheek wound closure.

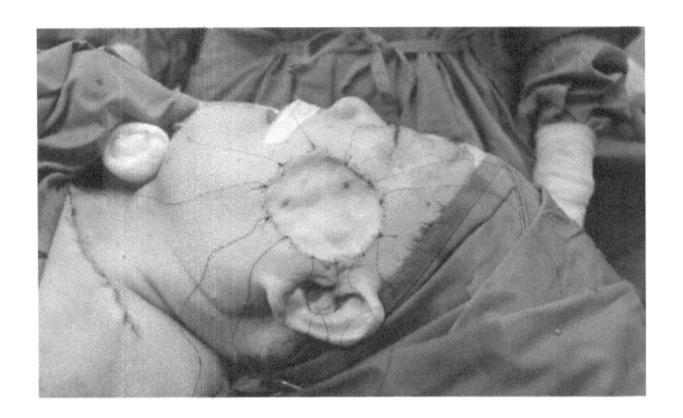

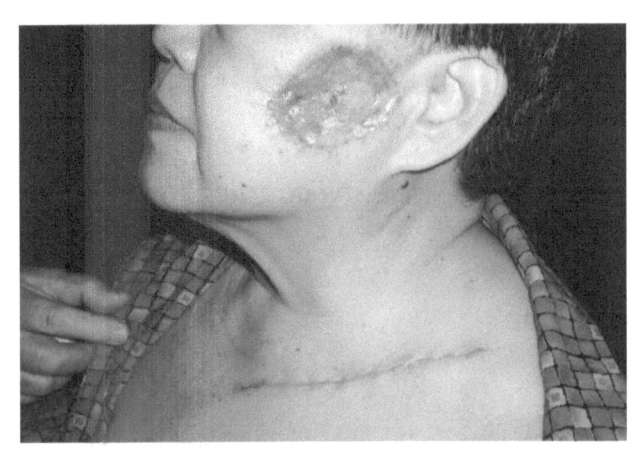

FTG is ideal for areas of face and joint surfaces. The size of FTG harvested is limited to a small size as the donor site is closed primarily.

Indication	
Flap is generally to cover a significant contour defect that may be exposing vital structures e.g. internal organ, bone, neurovascular bundle, implant, etc.	SSG is generally to cover large area of wound with healthy granulation tissue (without exposing vital structures) e.g. burn injury wounds, degloving injury wounds.

Example

1. Pressure wound closed with local flap.

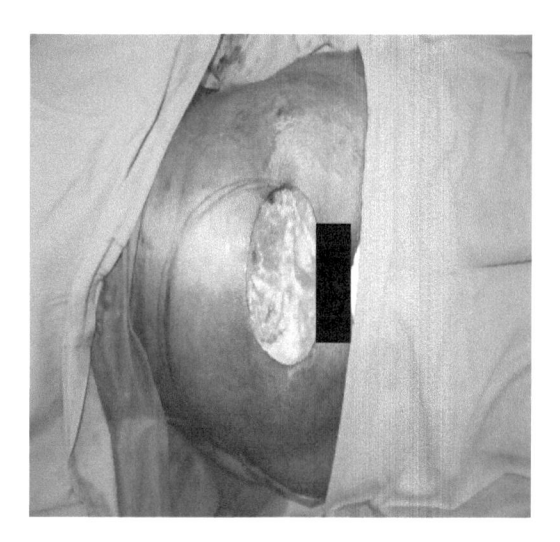

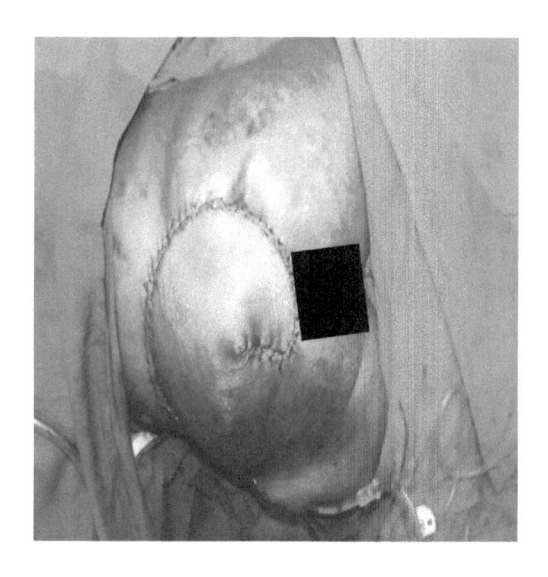

1. Burn wound closure with SSG

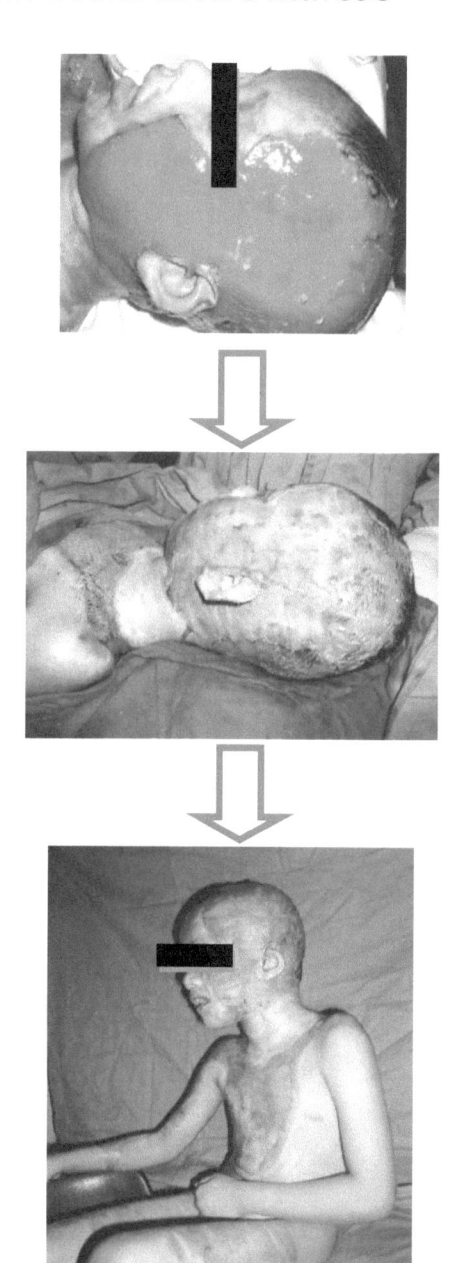

SECTION A: BASIC WOUND PRINCIPLE | 49

2. Complex wound after cancer extirpation exposing vital structures is closed with free fasciocutaneous flap.

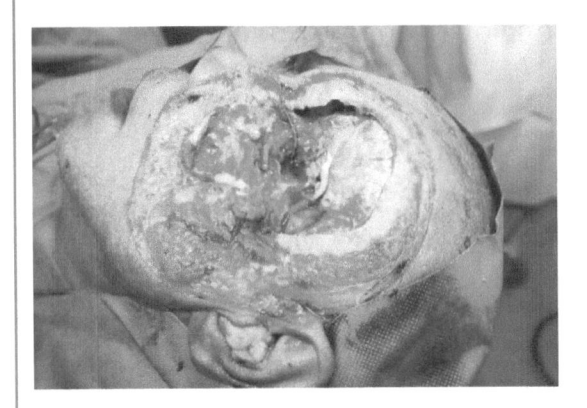

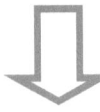

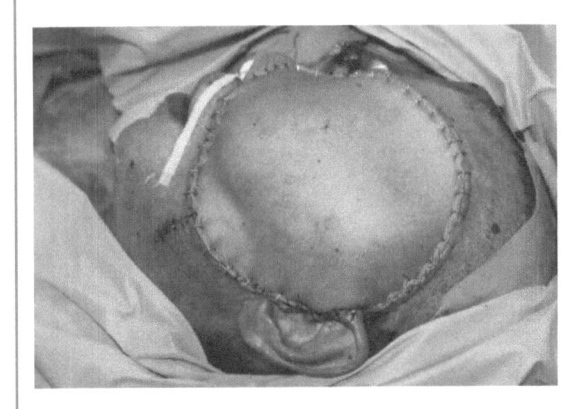

6-7. Tissue Expansion

Utilizing this modality for the primary closure of the particular wound may be limited due to the fact that the size, location, or zone of injury may preclude the use of adjacent tissue for expansion. However, tissue expansion does have a role at a secondary procedure. A wound may be treated with SSG initially to close the wound. The surrounding skin is then expanded at a secondary procedure for durable skin coverage, with correction of the resulting scar or contour deformity.

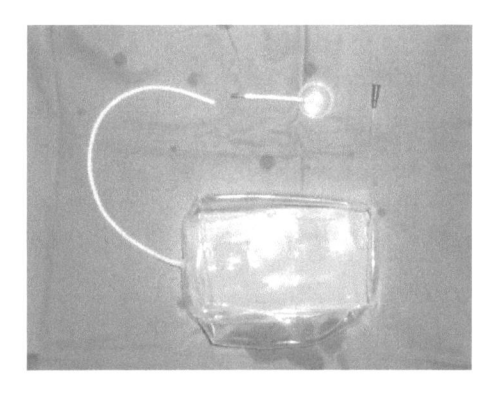

Figure 6.6 Tissue Expander

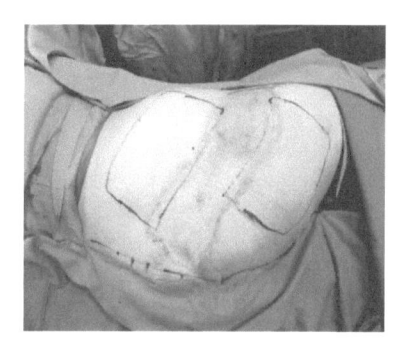

Figure 6.7 Post traumatic large soft tissue loss over the right gluteal region was skin grafted resulting in contour deformity and scar.

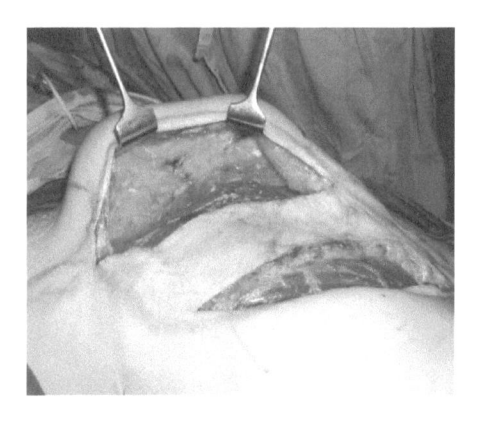

Subcutaneous pocket is created to insert the tissue expander

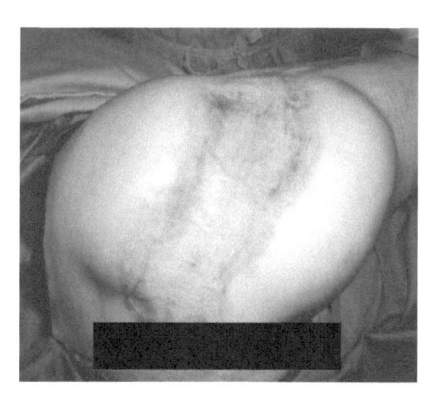

Periodical expansion till the desired volume achieved.

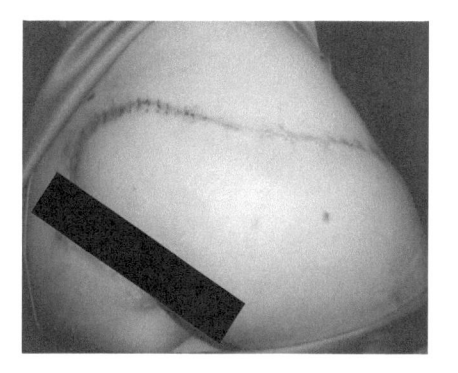

Skin grafted scar excised and expanded normal skin approximated hence closed primarily

SECTION A: BASIC WOUND PRINCIPLE | 51

Point to Remember:

- Healthy and stable wound is a prerequisite before wound closure.
- Options for wound closure must always ensure:
    - safe and successful surgery,
    - restoration of form and aesthetically acceptable
    - preservation of function
- Reconstructive ladder is a guide to wound closure.

References

1. Hansen, S. L., Mathes, S. J. *Problem wounds and Principles of closure. Plastic Surgery* 2nd ed. Saunders Elsevier, Philadelphia 2006.

2. Mathes, S. J., Nahai, F., *Reconstuctive Surgery: Principles, Anatomy, and Technique.* New York, Churchill Livingstone, 1997.

3. Jeffrey E. Janis, Robert K. Kwon, Christopher E. Attinger. *The New Reconstructive Ladder: Modifications to the Traditional Model.* PRS January Supplement 2011. 205s – 212s.

SECTION B:
Concept of Wound Care Management

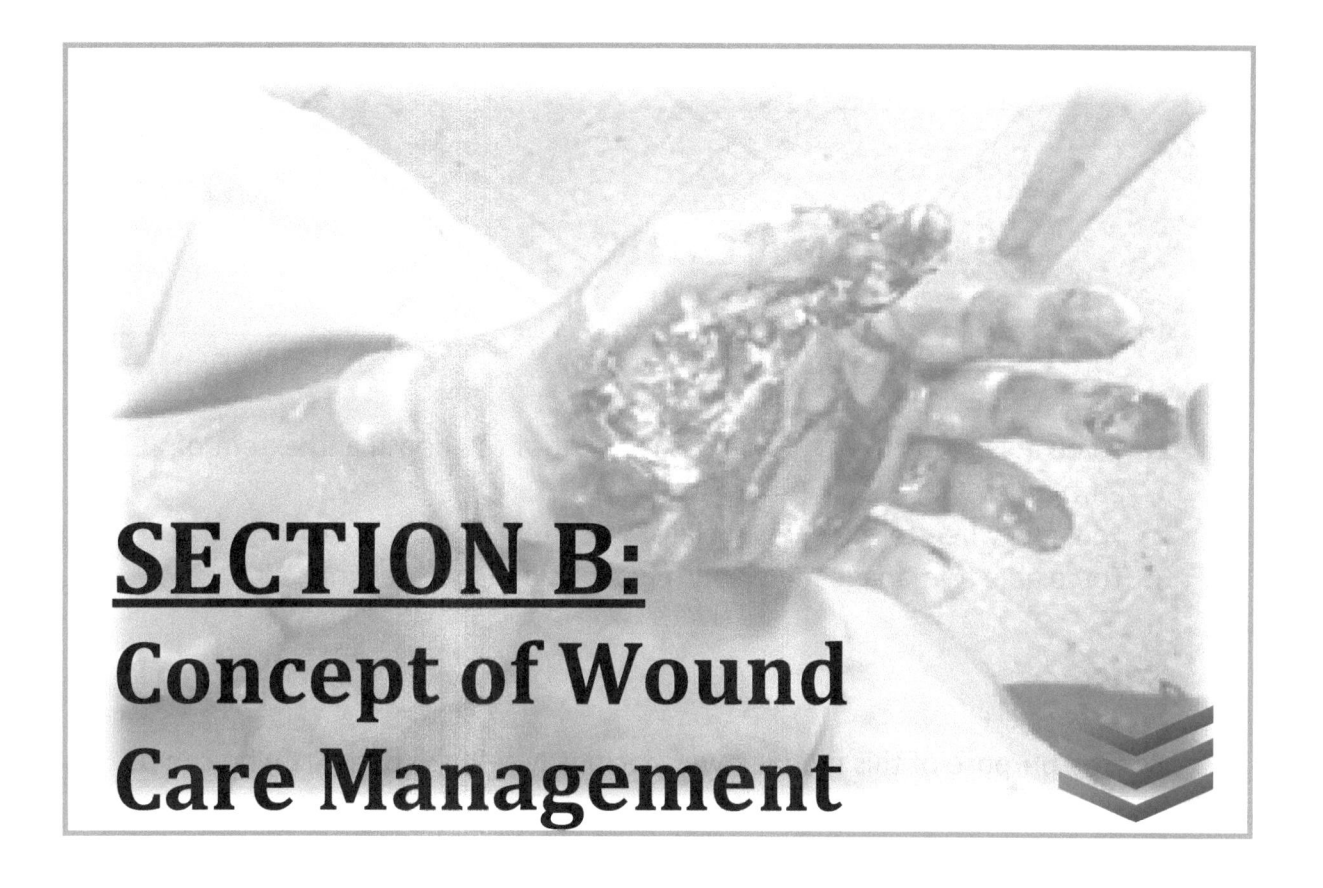

CHAPTER	TOPIC	CONTRIBUTORS

Chapter 7	Management of Acute Wound
	  a) Burn Wound
	  b) Traumatic Wound
		Dr Wu Loo Yee
		Dr Andre Das

Chapter 8	Management of Chronic Wound
	  a) Diabetic Foot ulcer
	  b) Venous and Arterial Ulcers
	  c) Pressure Ulcer
		Dr Mohammad Anwar Hau
		Dr Hanif
		Dr Zairizam/ Dr Khairiah

Chapter 9	Management of Non-Healing Ulcer	*Dr Andre Das*
Chapter 10	Management of Life-Threatening Wound	*Dr Mohammad Anwar Hau*
Chapter 11	Analgesia for Wound Dressing Related Procedures	*Dr Kavita/ Dr Mary Cardosa/ Dr Harijah*

CHAPTER 7

Management of Acute Wound
a) Burn Wound

Dr. Wu Loo Yee

AIMS:
1. To be able to perform correct assessment of the depth and extent of burn injury
2. To know when to refer to Specialist Hospital
3. To be able to manage minor burn wounds in a local setting

SCOPE:
For the purpose of this manual, we specifically refer to patients who can be managed in a non-specialized centre

7a-1. Introduction

Burn injury is a surgical emergency, which requires prompt and aggressive treatment. The management of burns requires a multi-disciplinary approach in order to obtain the best aesthetic and functional outcome.

The aim of modern burn management after the initial resuscitation is to achieve early wound closure and prevent burn sepsis. Early tangential excision and skin grafting is very important to prevent the occurrence of hypertrophic scarring and the resultant disabling contractures which are often difficult to treat and time consuming.

Causes of burn:
1. Thermal (flame)
2. Hot liquids (scalds)
3. Chemical (acids, alkalis, corrosives)
4. Electrical and lightning
5. Radiation
6. Inhalation
7. Friction (abrasion)

Depth of Burn Injury

Depending upon the depth of tissue damage, burns may be classified as either superficial or deep. In practice, all burns are a mixture of areas of different depth.

Table 7a.1 Diagnosis of Burn Depth

Epidermal (1st degree)	Partial thickness (2nd degree)		Full thickness (3rd degree)
	Superficial dermal	Deep dermal	
Colour			
Hyperemia	Pale pink	Blotchy red	White leathery
Blisters			
None	Present	Present	None
Capillary refill			
Present	Present	Absent	Absent
Sensation			
Very painful	Very painful	Absent	Absent
Spontaneous healing			
Yes	Yes	No	No
Physical Appearance			

* Patients with deep dermal and full thickness (3rd degree) burn require immediate referral to specialist hospital

7a-2. Management of the Burn Wound

1. Burn injury is a medical emergency. After immediate first aid has been given, the principles of primary and secondary survey and simultaneous resuscitation should be followed as per ATLS principles (Airway, Breathing, Circulation, Disability, Exposure, and Fluid Resuscitation).

2. The burn areas are assessed using the Lund and Browder chart Figure 7a-1. This will help to identify patients that need to be referred to a specialized medical facility (see Table 7a-2) and to start fluid resuscitation as per Parkland Formula.

A BURN CHART

NAME_____ WARD_____ NUMBER_____ DATE_____
AGE_____

LUND AND BROWDER CHARTS

Ignore simple erythema.

▨ Superficial
▨ Deep

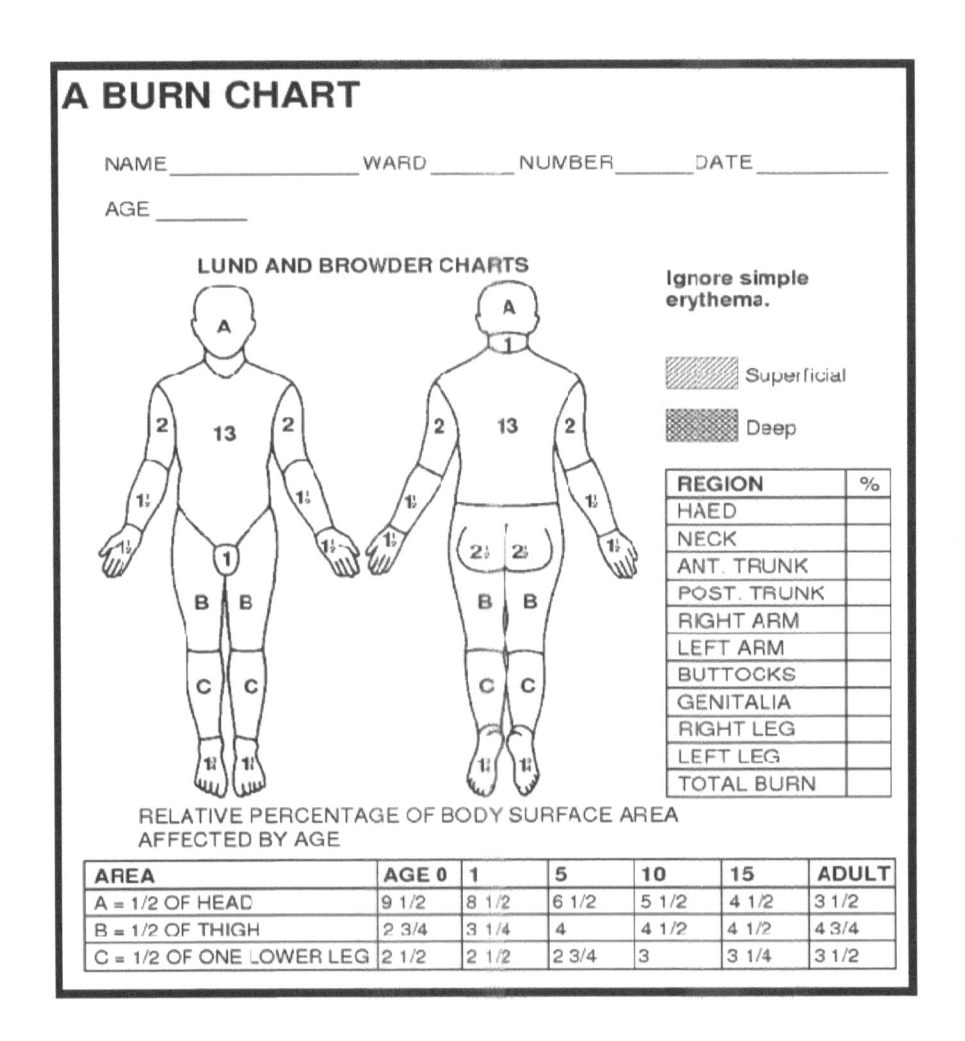

REGION	%
HAED	
NECK	
ANT. TRUNK	
POST. TRUNK	
RIGHT ARM	
LEFT ARM	
BUTTOCKS	
GENITALIA	
RIGHT LEG	
LEFT LEG	
TOTAL BURN	

RELATIVE PERCENTAGE OF BODY SURFACE AREA AFFECTED BY AGE

AREA	AGE 0	1	5	10	15	ADULT
A = 1/2 OF HEAD	9 1/2	8 1/2	6 1/2	5 1/2	4 1/2	3 1/2
B = 1/2 OF THIGH	2 3/4	3 1/4	4	4 1/2	4 1/2	4 3/4
C = 1/2 OF ONE LOWER LEG	2 1/2	2 1/2	2 3/4	3	3 1/4	3 1/2

Figure 7a.1 The Lund and Browder Chart
The Lund and Browder chart for the assessment of the total body surface area of burns (TBSA).
Note: areas of erythema are not included

Criteria for Injuries Requiring Referral to Specialist Hospital

1. Full thickness burns greater than 5% TBSA in any age group;
2. Partial thickness burns > 10% TBSA in patients in paediatric age groups and adult > 50 years of age;
3. Partial thickness burns > 15% TBSA in all groups;
4. Burns involving the face, hands, feet, genitalia, perineum and over joints;
5. Electrical burns, including lightning injury;
6. Chemical burns with serious functional and cosmetic impairment;
7. Suspicion of inhalational injury
8. Burn injury in patients with pre-existing medical disorders that could complicate management, prolong recovery or increase the mortality rate;
9. Any burn patient with concomitant trauma (e.g. fractures or intra-abdominal injuries);
10. Burn injury in patients who require special social, emotional, and/or long-term rehabilitative support, including cases of suspected child abuse, substance abuse, etc.

Adopted from American Burn Association Criteria for referral to Burn Center

3. In extensive burns, the appropriate treatment is to cover the wound with a clean sheet or plastic cling wrap before transfer. Do not cover the burns with Silver Sulfadiazine (SSD) as it may mask the depth of burns. Remember to keep the patient warm.

4. Cover minor burns with dressings such as paraffin gauze moistened with sterile normal saline or 0.1% aqueous chlorhexidine solution.

5. Do not constrict limb circulation with tight dressings. It is important to elevate the involved extremities.

6. Since burn injury is a wound, local protocol for tetanus must be followed.

7. Adequate pain relief must be provided (refer to chapter on pain management).

8. If the burns appear to be epidermal or superficial partial thickness, continue with either topical antimicrobial dressings (SSD), paraffin gauze or any available modern wound dressings until the wound heals (please refer to the chapter on wound dressing material).

9. If the burns are full thickness, or deep partial thickness which are unlikely to heal within 3 weeks, you may want to refer to a specialist hospital where patient may require tangential excision and split-thickness skin grafting (Figure 7a.2)

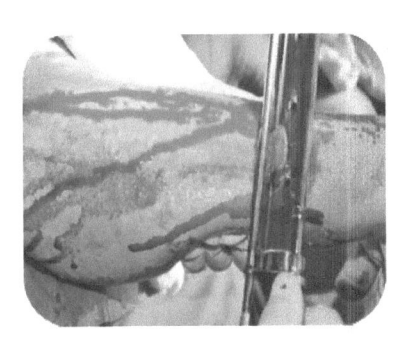

Figure 7a.2 Tangential excision of partial thickness burn wound until viable tissue.

10. There is no need for prophylactic antibiotics unless there is evidence of infection.

11. Remember the importance of splinting the affected joints to prevent contractures. Patient must continue with rehabilitation upon discharge.

12. The use of pressure garments may continue for up to one year or two depending on the severity of the hypertrophic scarring.

13. All patients must be followed up for at least six months to one year to detect any developing contractures and hypertrophic scars which warrants a referral to a plastic surgeon.

Indications for Referral to Specialist Hospital after Failure of Conservative Management

i. No progress of healing after 3 weeks of treatment.

ii. Presence of slough, necrotic patch or infection.

iii. Occurrence of hypertrophic scarring and early contractures.

Points to remember

- Know how to assess severity of burn injury
- Know when to refer to Specialist Hospital

References

1. Rajiv Sood, Bruce M Achauer. Achauer and Sood's Burn Surgery: Reconstruction and Rehabilitation: Elsevier: 50-76; 2006.

2. John L Hunt, Gary F Purdue, Ross I S Zbar. Burns: Acute Burns, Burn Surgery, And Postburn Reconstruction. Selected Readings in Plastic Surgery 9(12), 2000.

3. Jeffrey J Roth, William B Hughes. The Essential Burn Unit Handbook: Quality Medical Publishing; 2004.

4. Greenfield LJ, Mulholland M, Oldham KT, Zelenock GB, Lillemoe KD. Surgery, Scientific Principles and Practice, 2nd ed. Philadelphia: Lippincott-Raven, 1997.

CHAPTER 7

Management of Acute Wound
b) Traumatic Wound

Dr Andre Das

AIM:
To achieve wound healing in the quickest possible manner with minimal morbidity and best cosmetic results

SCOPE:
Wounds caused by trauma

7b-1. Clinical Assessment

History

Main Points:
- Time elapsed since injury
- Mechanism of injury
- Cleanliness of wound and possibility of retained foreign body
- AMPLE (Allergy, Medication, Past History, Last Meal, Environment)

Examination

a. Inspection
- Anatomical location and possibility of associated more serious injuries (especially neck, chest, abdomen)
- Size wound edge and tissue loss
- Cleanliness
- Viability

b. Palpation
- Crepitus or foreign bodies
- Neurovascular status
- Tendons and movement

Investigations

X-ray if indicated for possible foreign bodies or suspected bone fracture

7b-2. Treatment

Principles

1. Treat life or limb threatening conditions first

2. Initial management of the patient is as per ATLS principles.

3. Wounds which are bleeding torrentially and/or will lead to circulatory distress are included under the ATLS principles. All other wounds will be treated expectantly after settling primary survey conditions.

Management of Bleeding Wounds in Primary Survey

1. Stop bleeding in the fastest and simplest manner first rather than closure of the wound especially if other life threatening conditions are present.

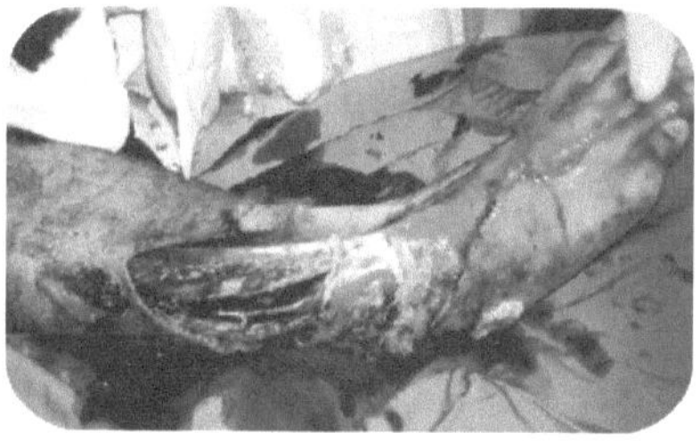

2. Options to stop bleeding include:

    ➢ direct pressure compression

    ➢ haemostatic sutures

    Figure 7b.1 Bleeding wound post trauma

    ➢ Tourniquet for special situations (controversial and to be applied with a specialist consult)

    ➢ Artery forceps especially for scalp wounds or laceration involving major vessels e.g. limb vessels.

    ➢ Haemostatic materials if available (expensive)

Local or General Anaesthesia

Dependent upon site and size of wounds, allergic constraints, patient factors e.g. age or patient's preference.

Toilet and debridement

1. Thorough irrigation with normal saline (refer respective chapter: cleansing solution)

2. Remove foreign materials and dirt

3. Debride unhealthy tissue

Primary closure

1. Aim for this in all cases if possible

2. Tension free closure

3. Possible methods include:

    ➢ Suture

    ➢ Skin adhesive strip

    ➢ Skin glue

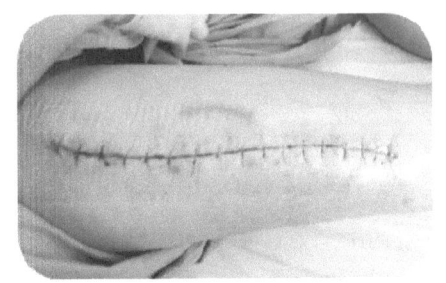

Figure 7b.2 Surgical wound closure with suture

Delayed Primary Closure

1. Definition: closure of the wound after 72-hour

2. Usually for the following conditions:

    - Minimal tissue loss
    - Dirty wounds e.g. bites, contaminated environment
    - More than 12 hours from time of injury

Secondary healing

When there is ext   tissue loss with inability to oppose wound edges and allow healing by granulation

Dressings

Any barrier dressing available that does not stick to the wound and has some adsorbent properties (refer to chapter on dressing materials)

Advice on discharge

- Keep wound dry, shower allowed after 48 hours but avoid soaking wounds
- Avoid getting wound dirty
- Avoid exposure to direct sunlight especially for facial wounds
- Dressing may be removed after 48 hours
- Seek medical help if wound is foul smelling, there is extreme pain or extensive discharge
- Date for removal of sutures if used. Otherwise can allow glue and skin adhesive strip to drop off by itself or after wound healed visually

7b-3. Precautions

Special Situations Which May Need Specialist Consult / referral

- Facial wounds especially to eyelid, ear, Vermillion border of lip
- Suspected nerve or tendon injury
- Deep wounds in areas e.g. neck, chest, abdomen
- Joints
- Electrical or severe crush injuries

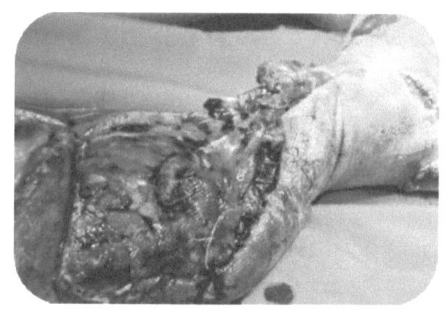

Figure 7b.3 Crush injury of the leg following motor vehicle accident

Cases which need close follow up after primary closure

- Infection prone area e.g. perineum
- Degloving injuries where viability may be suspect
- Pedicled wounds where viability may be suspect especially with narrow base
- Patients with significant co-morbid e.g. Diabetes, immunocompromised conditions, malnourished, on medications which may impair healing e.g. steroids, chemotherapy
- Wound infected after primary closure should be opened up, drained and dressed and let it heal by secondary intention. Antibiotic might be considered.

7b-3. Adjuncts

1. Antibiotics: In the wound context generally not needed, except for a possible single prophylactic dose before primary closure. No substitute for surgery. Exceptions where empirical antibiotics may be needed include:
    i. Communication with bone fractures or joint space
    ii. Areas with difficulty in adequate debridment e.g. near tendons and fascial spaces of hands
    iii. Delayed treatment >6 hours
    iv. Involving entry into a hollow viscus organ esp GIT
    v. Immunocompromised patients
    vi. Clostridial prone wounds soil contamination wound

2. Choice of antibiotic → refer National Antibiotic Guidelines

3. Antitetanus: according to local protocol

4. Splints : for immobilisation in special situations

5. Colostomy for certain perineal wounds

6. Continous bladder drainage when indicated

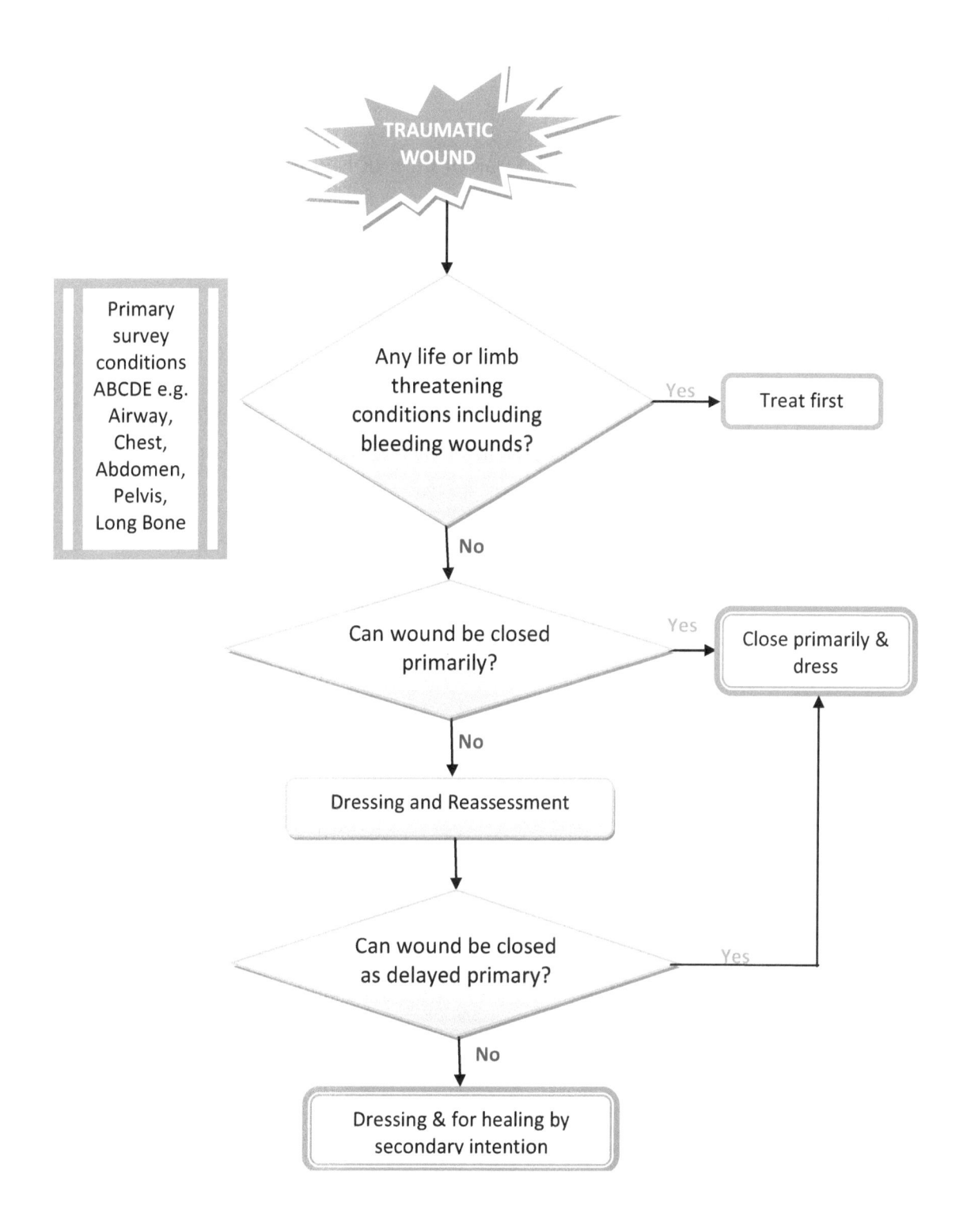

```
                    TRAUMATIC
                     WOUND
                        │
                        ▼
┌──────────────┐   ╱ Any life or limb ╲
│   Primary    │  ╱    threatening     ╲   Yes   ┌─────────────┐
│   survey     │ ╱  conditions including ╲──────▶│ Treat first │
│  conditions  │ ╲   bleeding wounds?    ╱       └─────────────┘
│  ABCDE e.g.  │  ╲                     ╱
│   Airway,    │   ╲                   ╱
│    Chest,    │       │ No
│   Abdomen,   │       ▼
│    Pelvis,   │   ╱ Can wound be closed ╲   Yes   ┌──────────────────┐
│   Long Bone  │  ╱      primarily?       ╲───────▶│ Close primarily &│
└──────────────┘  ╲                       ╱       │      dress       │
                   ╲                     ╱        └──────────────────┘
                        │ No                              ▲
                        ▼                                 │
                 ┌─────────────────────────┐              │
                 │ Dressing and Reassessment│             │
                 └─────────────────────────┘              │
                        │                                 │
                        ▼                                 │
                   ╱ Can wound be closed ╲   Yes          │
                  ╱  as delayed primary?  ╲───────────────┘
                   ╲                     ╱
                        │ No
                        ▼
                 ┌──────────────────────────┐
                 │ Dressing & for healing by│
                 │   secondary intention    │
                 └──────────────────────────┘
```

Figure 7b.4 Algorithm for management of traumatic wound

> **Points to remember**
> - All traumatic wounds have risk of infection

References

1. *Adam J. Singer, M.D., Judd E. Hollander, M.D., and James V. Quinn, M.D. N. Evaluation and Management of Traumatic Lacerations Engl J Med 1997; 337:1142-1148*

CHAPTER 8

Management of Chronic Wound
a) Diabetic Foot Ulcer

Dr Mohammad Anwar Hau Abdullah

8a-1. Introduction

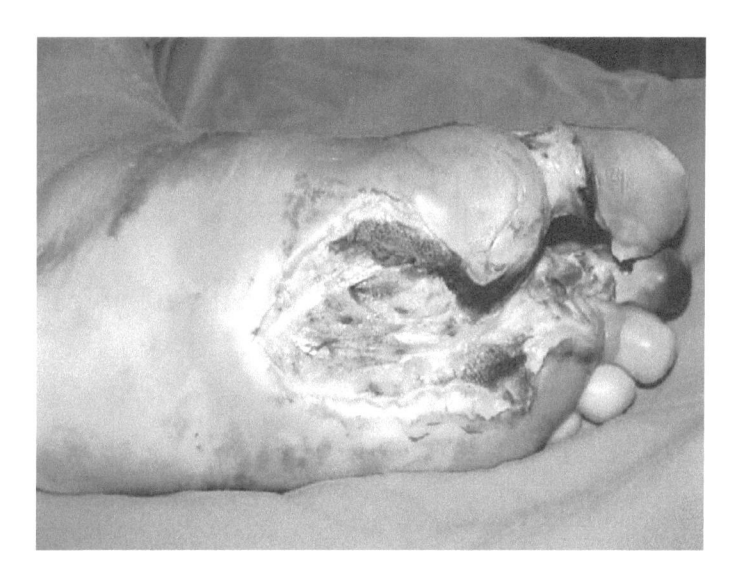

Figure 8a.1 Diabetic foot Ulcer

- Diabetic foot is a foot that exhibits any pathology that results directly from diabetes mellitus or any long-term (or "chronic") complication of diabetes mellitus (Jeffcoate & Harding, 2003).

- Diabetic foot implies that the pathophysiological process of diabetes mellitus does something to the foot that puts it at increased risk for "tissue damage" and the resultant increase in morbidity and maybe amputation (Payne & Florkowski, 1998).

Incidence of Diabetic Foot Ulcer

- Studies have indicated that diabetic patients have up to a 25% lifetime risk of developing a foot ulcer.

- The annual incidence of diabetic foot ulcers is ~ 3% to as high as 10%. (Armstrong and Lavery, 1998)

Pathophysiology of Diabetic Foot Ulcer

Diabetic are prone to foot ulceration due to:

- Neuropathy- leads to skin dryness and cracks, foot deformity and loss of protective sense in the foot
- Microangiopathy/vascular disease- lead to poor blood supply to the toes and foot and then ulcerate easily
- Immunopathy- Defects in leukocyte function (leukocyte phagocytosis, neutrophil dysfunction) and also deficient white cell chemotaxis and adherence

Clinical Presentation

- Soft tissue infections (superficial to deep tissue infection e.g. cellulitis, necrotizing fasciitis, etc.)
- Osteomyelitis (bone infection)
- Septic arthritis (joint infection)
- Gangrene (dry or wet)
- Chronic non-healing ulcer
- Combination of more than one of the above mentioned condition

8a-2. Assessment of Diabetic Foot Ulcer

1. **History:**
   - Diabetic history
   - Previous ulcer or amputation
   - Symptoms of peripheral neuropathy
   - Symptoms of peripheral vascular/ischemic problem
   - Contributing factors

- Other complications of diabetes (eyes, kidney, heart etc).
- Current ulcer

2. **Examination:**

Thorough and carefully examine the whole foot for the following:-

- Previous amputation/ulcer
- Deformity and footwear
- Inspect web spaces - signs of infection or wound
- Hypercallosity or nail deformity or paronychia
- Present of peripheral neuropathy with tuning folks, also monofilament and position sense.
- Peripheral pulses - peripheral vascular disease
- Ankle-brachial index (ABSI)
- Other relevant systems (renal, eye, heart etc)

Do not forget to examine the other foot!

8a-3. Classification of Diabetic Foot Ulcer

Wagner Classification of Diabetic Foot Ulcers (more commonly used)

Grade	Description
0	No ulcer in a high risk foot (callosities, deformity, skin dryness etc)
1	Superficial ulcer involving the partial or full skin thickness but not underlying tissues.
2	Deep ulcer, penetrating down to ligaments and muscle, but no bone involvement or abscess formation.
3	Deep ulcer with cellulitis or abscess formation, often with osteomyelitis or joint sepsis.
4	Localized gangrene (portion of forefoot or heel).
5	Extensive gangrene involving the whole foot

8a-4. Clinical Photos of Diabetic Foot Ulcer

Wagner 0: Foot at risk

Wagner 0: Foot at risk: deformity secondary to neuropathic joint

Wagner 0: Foot at risk: previous amputation and deformity

Wagner Grade 1: superficial skin infection (cellulitis)

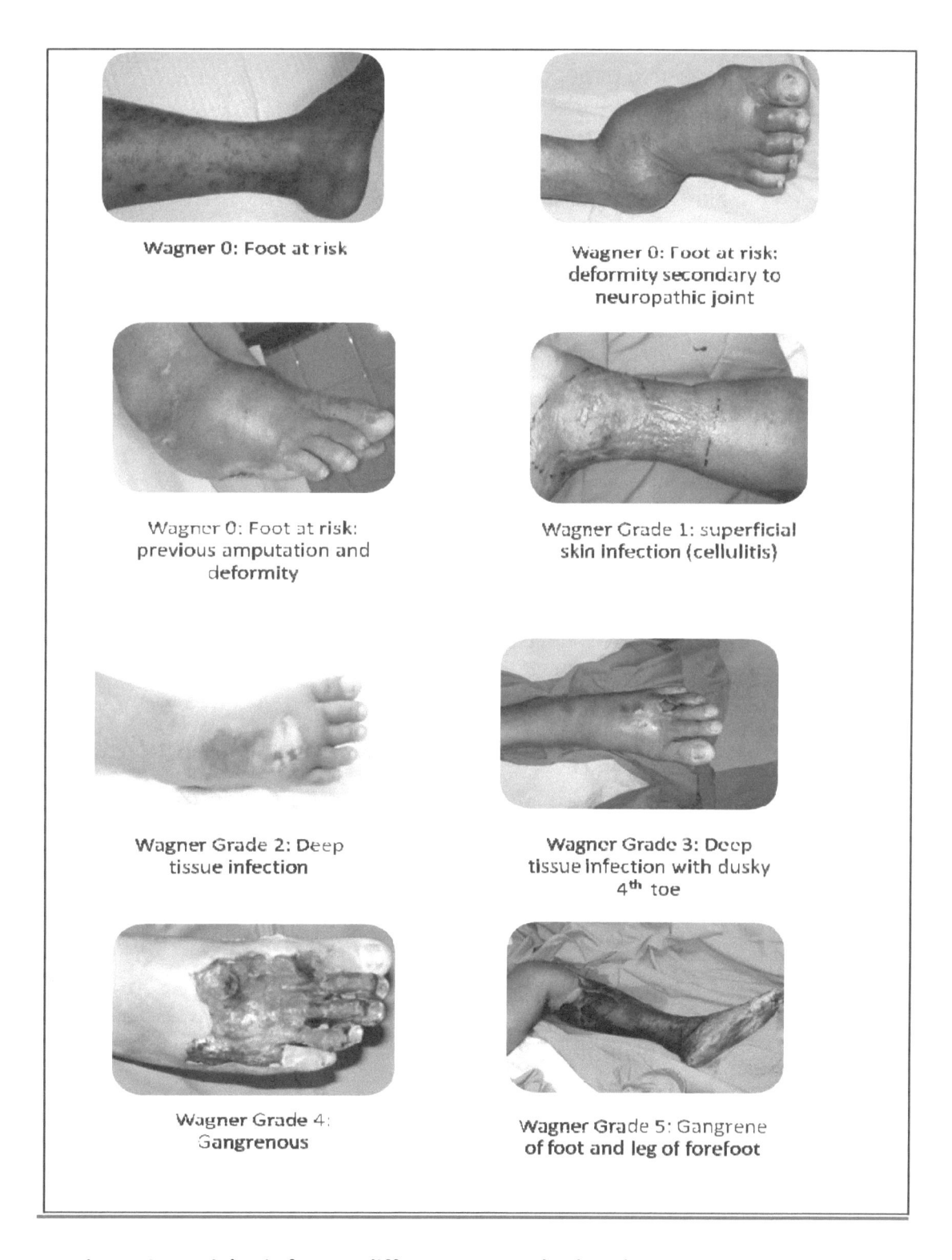

Wagner Grade 2: Deep tissue infection

Wagner Grade 3: Deep tissue infection with dusky 4th toe

Wagner Grade 4: Gangrenous

Wagner Grade 5: Gangrene of foot and leg of forefoot

Figure 8a.2 Diabetic foot at different Wagner's Classification

Foot at risk of ulceration

- History of ulceration
- Presence of neuropathy
- Presence of peripheral vascular disease
- Presence of foot deformity
- Inappropriate footwear
- Skin lesion
- Nail pathology
- Duration of diabetes
- Prolonged standing or walking
- Type of occupation

8a-5. Management of Diabetic Foot Ulcer

Objective:
- Control infection
- Ulcer/wound management
- Prevent amputation
- Maintain pre-morbid foot/lower extremity function as much as possible
- Prevent recurrent ulcer

1. *General management:*
   - A multidisciplinary approach
   - Good diabetic control
   - Systemic antibiotics (according to CPG on Antibiotic Guideline and also culture and sensitivity of the infected tissue)
   - Optimise other co-morbid complications.
   - Advise to stop smoking

2. *Local management:*

- Wound/ulcer management: depending on severity of wound; vascularity and also presence of infection.
- .Debride infected/necrotic tissue follow by wound management (refer Wound care Algorithm in Chapter 17)
- Do not hesitate to perform re-debridement if indicated.
- Amputation may be the treatment of choice.
- Minimize risk of re-infection
- If indicated reestablished adequate blood supply (refer to chapter on arterial ulcer).
- Off loading with contact cast etc (Appendix 2).
- Good foot care and foot wear (Appendix 3)

If no signs of healing after 2 weeks of treatment, reevaluate and looks for the cause.

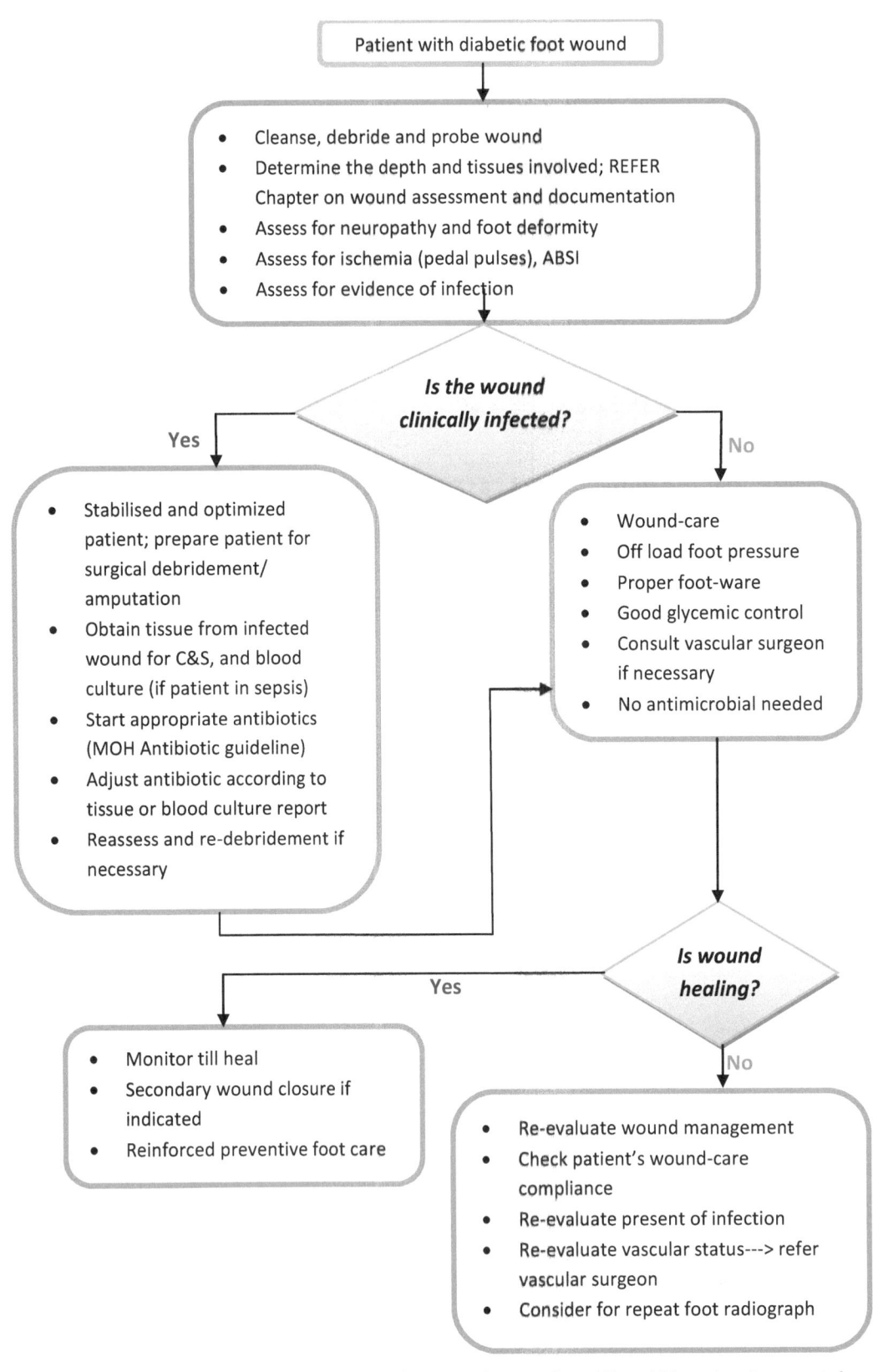

```
                    ┌─────────────────────────────┐
                    │ Patient with diabetic foot wound │
                    └─────────────┬───────────────┘
                                  ▼
    ┌──────────────────────────────────────────────────────────┐
    │ • Cleanse, debride and probe wound                       │
    │ • Determine the depth and tissues involved; REFER        │
    │   Chapter on wound assessment and documentation          │
    │ • Assess for neuropathy and foot deformity               │
    │ • Assess for ischemia (pedal pulses), ABSI               │
    │ • Assess for evidence of infection                       │
    └──────────────────────────┬───────────────────────────────┘
                               ▼
                    ╱╲ Is the wound ╱╲
             Yes  ╱    clinically infected?  ╲  No
                 ╱                             ╲
```

- Stabilised and optimized patient; prepare patient for surgical debridement/amputation
- Obtain tissue from infected wound for C&S, and blood culture (if patient in sepsis)
- Start appropriate antibiotics (MOH Antibiotic guideline)
- Adjust antibiotic according to tissue or blood culture report
- Reassess and re-debridement if necessary

- Wound-care
- Off load foot pressure
- Proper foot-ware
- Good glycemic control
- Consult vascular surgeon if necessary
- No antimicrobial needed

Is wound healing?

Yes →
- Monitor till heal
- Secondary wound closure if indicated
- Reinforced preventive foot care

No →
- Re-evaluate wound management
- Check patient's wound-care compliance
- Re-evaluate present of infection
- Re-evaluate vascular status---> refer vascular surgeon
- Consider for repeat foot radiograph

Reference: Lipsky BA, Berendt AR, Deery HG, Embil JM, Joseph WS, Karchmer AW, et al. Diagnosis and treatment of diabetic foot infections. Clin Infect Dis 2004;39:889.

Figure 8a.2 Treatment Algorithm of a Patient with a Diabetic Foot Wound

Diabetic foot-care

- Foot inspection- minimally once a day
- Use lukewarm (*air suam*), not hot water to wash feet
- Use gentle soap to bath/wash feet
- Apply moisturizer to avoid dry feet – be careful with the web space and not too much (causing skin maceration)
- Proper nail cutting, avoid cutting too close/digging nail fold.
- Wear clean, dry socks (NEVER use heating pad or hot water bottle) to keep foot warm
- Avoid walk barefooted.
- Wear comfortable well fitting shoe (not too tight or too loose), evening is the best time to buy shoe. Refer to Foot Care in Appendix 3
- Shake out shoes and feel the inside before wearing
- Never treat corns or calluses themselves
- Good diabetic control
- Stop smoking
- Periodic foot examination by relevant personals
- Keep the blood flowing to feet (elevate, wiggers toes, moving ankle) , avoid cross-leg or hanging leg/feet too long

Point to remember:

- Good glycemic control, regular foot assessment; including vascular and neurological assessment; to prevent diabetic foot ulcer.
- The main underlying cause of diabetic foot ulcer is chronic pressure- think of off loading.
- Diabetic foot ulcer need multidisciplinary approach

References

1. *James Teh, Tony Berendt, Benjamin A Lipsky. Investigating suspected bone infection in the diabetic foot. BMJ 2009;339:b4690.*

2. *Warren Clayton, Jr.Tom A. Elasy.* **A Review of the Pathophysiology, Classification, and Treatment of Foot Ulcers in Diabetic Patients.** Clinical Diabetes *Spring 2009 vol. 27 no. 252-58.*

3. **Armstrong DG. And Lavery LA. Diabetic Foot Ulcers: Prevention, Diagnosis and Classification.** *Am Fam. Physician. 1998 Mar 15; 57(6):1325-1332.*

4. Frykberg RG. Diabetic Foot Ulcers: Pathogenesis and Management. Am Fam. Physician. 2002 Nov 1; 66(9):1655-1663.

Management of Chronic Wound
b) Venous Ulcer

Dr Hanif Hussein

8b-1. Introduction

Venous ulcer is the commonest cause of leg ulcer and it contributes to a significant socio-economic disability in the population as it affects the quality of life. It is due to presence of venous hypertension in the lower limbs.

8b-2. Classification

There are two major groups of venous ulcer, with different treatment options and outcomes.

1. **Ulcer secondary to primary varicose veins**

    - In this group of patients, treating the varicosities will usually result in ulcer healing.

2. **Ulcer secondary to deep venous incompetence**

    - Post-phlebitic syndromes contribute to a big proportion of this group and treatment is aimed to improve healing rate and reducing recurrence of the ulcer.

8b-3. Risk Factors and Associated Factors

Risk factors for chronic venous ulcer:

1. Varicose veins
2. Deep vein thrombosis
3. Chronic venous insufficiency
4. Poor calf muscle function
5. Obesity
6. History of leg injury
7. Family history

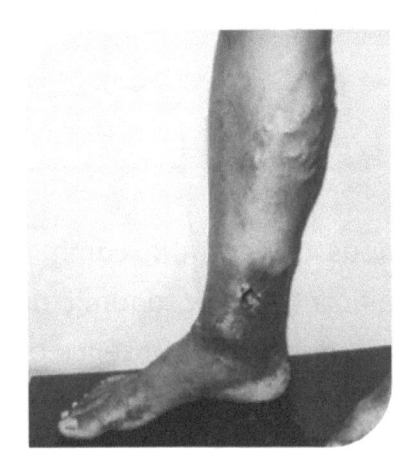

Figure 8b.1 Venous ulcer over the Gaiter's area

Associated factors:

1. Diabetes mellitus
2. Heart failure
3. Hypertension
4. Renal disease
5. Rheumatoid arthritis

8b-4. Diagnosis

Diagnosis of venous ulcer is made based on history and physical examination.

History:
1. Risk factors
    - Above listed risk factors should be identified

2. History of deep vein thrombosis
    - Documented or suggestive history of previous DVT

3. Symptoms of chronic venous insufficiency
    - Calf heaviness after prolonged standing

Examination:
1. Examination of the ulcer/wound
    - Typical site: just above the medial malleolus – the Gaiter's area.
    - Leg edema, thickening and hyperpigmentation (lipodermatosclerosis) of the surrounding skin.

2. Varicose veins
    - May or may not be present. These may just be telengeactasia, spider veins or varicosities along the long or short saphenous veins

3. Peripheral arterial pulses
    - Palpate and confirm distal pulses to exclude arterial disease

8b-5. Investigations

A duplex ultrasound scan is required in patients suspected to have ulcer secondary to deep venous incompetence

- To look for deep vein patency and incompetence
- To identify sapheno-femoral or sapheno-popliteal junction incompetence
- To identify and localize incompetent perforators

8b-6. Treatment

Leg elevation and compression bandaging are the most important components of treatment. It is **crucial to exclude peripheral arterial disease** before commencing on compression therapy.

1. Elevation of the leg
   - Reduces leg edema and promote wound healing
   - Elevate higher than the heart level

2. Graduated compression stockings and compression bandages
   - Multi-layer compression (4 layer or 2 layer) is used during the acute phase
   - Graduated compression stockings can be used once the wound is more dry

3. For local management of a venous ulcer refer to Wound Care Algorithm in Chapter 17

4. In cases of venous ulcer secondary to primary varicose veins, patients should be referred for surgical intervention with high saphenous vein ligation once the acute phase and infection is under control.

5. Pharmacotherapy
   - Venotonic agents, e.g. Micronised flavinoids aids in the venous flow
   - Hemorheologic agents, e.g. Pentoxifylline

Four Layer Compression Bandage

	Material	Function
First layer	Orthopedic wool	Adsorbs exudate Redistribute pressure
Second layer	Cotton crepe bandage	Further adsorb exudate Smoothen orthopedic wool layer
Third layer	Elastic, extensible bandage (20 – 40 mmHg)	First layer of elastic compression
Fourth layer	Cohesive bandage	Second layer of elastic compression

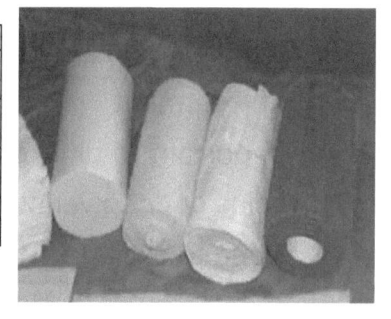

The first and second layers being applied

The third and fourth layers being applied

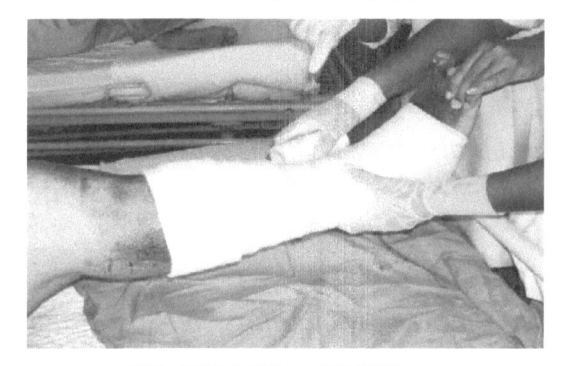

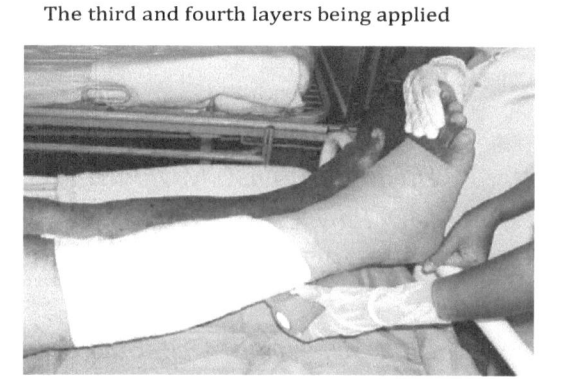

Figure 8b.2 Four-layer compression bandage

6. Pharmacotherapy
   - Venotonic agents, e.g. Micronised flavinoids aids in the venous flow
   - Hemorheologic agents, e.g. Pentoxifylline

7. Life-style modification to reduce rate of recurrence
   - Change of work
   - Weight reduction and dietary counseling

Conclusion

Venous ulcer is one of the common causes of le.g. ulcer and it causes a significant socio-economic disability. It is crucial to identify ulcers that are due to primary varicose veins for surgical intervention. Otherwise, treatment involves a long-term management plan aimed to hasten healing and reduce recurrence.

> **Points to remember:**
>
> - Leg elevation and compression therapy are two important components of treatment
> - Important to differentiate between ulcer secondary to primary varicose veins or deep venous incompetence
> - Need to exclude arterial disease before commencing treatment

References

1. David Bergqvist, MD, PhD, Christina Lindholm, RN, PhD, and Olle Nelzén MD, PhD. Chronic leg ulcers: The impact of venousdisease. J Vasc Surg 1999;29:752-5.

2. Blair SD, Wright DDI, Backhouse CM, Riddle E, McCollum CN. Sustained compression and healing of chronic venous ulcers. BMJ 1988;297:1159-61

3. Maria T. Szewczyk et.al. Comparison of the effectiveness of compression stockings and layer compression systems in venous ulceration treatment. Arch Med Sci 2010; 6, 5: 793-799

4. Michael S. Weingarten. State-of-the-Art Treatment of Chronic Venous Disease. Clinical Infectious Diseases 2001; 32:949–54

5. Lyseng-Williamson KA, Perry CM. Micronised purified flavonoid fraction: a review of its use in chronic venous insufficiency, venous ulcers and haemorrhoids. Drugs. 2003;63(1):71-100

CHAPTER 8

Management of Chronic Wound
c) Arterial Ulcer

Dr Hanif Hussein/ Dr Khairiah Mohd Yatim

8c-1. Introduction

Arterial ulcers are ischemic ulcers in patients with peripheral vascular disease. Reduced blood supply to the affected limb impedes healing and causes delay or non-healing of the ulcer. It is crucial to identify arterial ulcers, as the management would involve revascularization to improve the circulation of the affected limb to achieve wound healing.

8c-2. Risk Factors

Risk factors for chronic limb ischemia include:

1. Diabetes mellitus
2. Smoking
3. Dyslipidemia
4. Male
5. Elderly
6. Hypertension
7. Hyperviscosity and hypercoaguable states

8c-3. Diagnosis

Diagnosis of arterial ulcer is based on history and physical examination.

Relevant History:
1. Risk factors.
   - Identify the above listed risk factors.

1. Symptoms of chronic limb ischemia.
   - Intermittent claudication – pain in the calf muscles with exercise and relieved by rest.
   - Rest pain – persistent pain (critical limb ischemia)

2. History of previous minor or major amputation
   - A patient with previous major amputation on the contra-lateral limb requires more aggressive efforts to salvage the currently affected limb

3. History of previous vascular intervention
   - A non-healing or recurrent wound indicates re-stenosis or thrombosis of previous intervention

5. Non-healing of a previous minor or major amputation wound.

Clinical Examination:

1. Examination of the ulcer/wound
   - Pale base and edges with slough
   - Void of granulation tissue
   - Dry ulcer with surrounding inflammation
   - Sites – Pressure points, toes

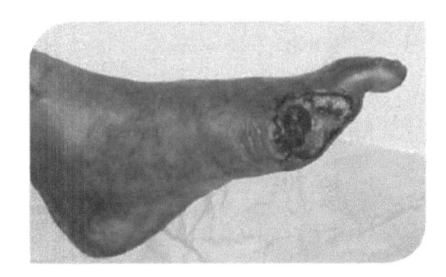

Figure 8c.1 Left foot arterial ulcer

2. Signs of chronic limb ischaemia
   - Muscle atrophy of the affected limb
   - Hair loss and hyperpigmentation

1. Examination of the peripheral pulses
   Digital palpation of the peripheral pulses.
   - Two plus (++) indicates normal pulse
   - One plus (+) indicates weak pulse
   - Negative (-) indicates absent pulse

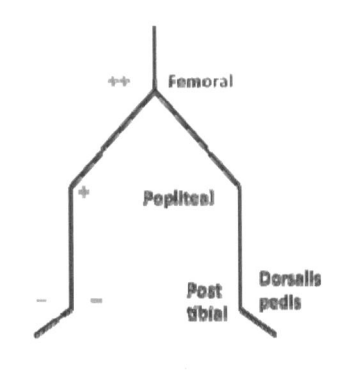

Documentation of digital palpation

2. Examination with a hand-held Doppler device

Waveform	ABSI	Interpretation
Triphasic	≥0.9 – 1.3	Normal
Biphasic	0.4 – 0.9	Peripheral vascular disease
Monophasic	≤ 0.4	Critical limb ischaemia

Note that ABSI may be normal or high with calcified vessels as in diabetic and some renal failure patients.

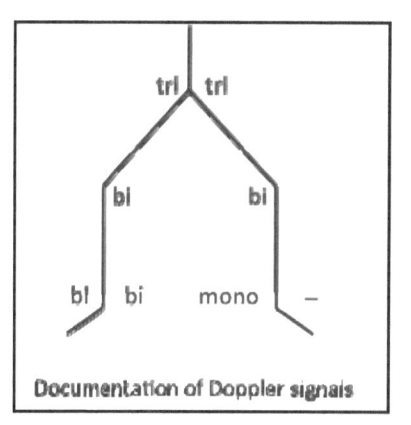

Documentation of Doppler signals

- Waveform of the Doppler signals and measurement of the ankle-brachial systolic index (ABSI) gives an indication of the severity of the disease in the vessels.

3. Toe pressure measurement (when available)
   - In patients with calcified vessels, where the ABSI maybe normal or high, toe pressure measurement would be more accurate to indicate presence or absence of peripheral vascular disease.

8c-4. Investigations

Non-healing ulcers with absent pulses or abnormal ABSI require radiological imaging to establish the level of disease and to plan subsequent intervention. Imaging options available includes duplex ultrasound scan, CT angiography, MR angiography and DS angiography. Choice of investigation depends on availability and suitability. Foot X-ray may be indicated to exclude underlying osteomyelitis

8c-5. Treatment

1. Re-vascularisation of diseased vessel
   - To restore/improve the circulation to the distal ischaemic limb
   - Can be achieved via open bypass surgery, angioplasty or in combination

2. Wound debridement / minor amputation and wound care
   - Following revascularization, standard wound care procedures as in Wound Care Algorithm in Chapter 17
   - Special care to be taken to avoid compression bandages and leg elevation

3. Pharmacotherapy
   - Anti-platelet therapy
   - Statins
   - Antibiotics when indicated
   - Analgesia (refer chapter on pain management)

4. Life-style modification
   - Stop smoking
   - Diabetic control
   - Dietary counseling

5. Major amputation
   - Primary amputation to be considered in non-salvageable limb, or patients with non-re-constructible disease and patients with poor cardiac function

6. Rehabilitation
   - Aim of treatment is for patients to ambulate and resume daily activities

Table 8c.1 Phases of amputee rehabilitation

1. Pre-operative	Medical and body condition assessment, patient education, surgical-level discussion, functional expectations, phantom limb discussion
2. Amputation surgery/dressing	Residual-limb length determination, myoplastic closure, soft-tissue coverage, nerve handling, rigid dressing application, limb reconstruction
3. Acute postsurgical	Wound healing, pain control, proximal body motion, emotional support, phantom limb discussion
4. Pre-prosthetic	Residual-limb shaping, shrinking, increasing muscle strength, restoring patient's sense of control (figure of 8 stump bandaging)
5. Prosthetic prescription/fabrication	Prosthetic prescription will depend on patient cognitive status, medical status, functional status and socioeconomic status
6. Prosthetic training	Prosthetic management and training to increase wearing time and functional use
7. Community integration	Resumption of family and community roles; regaining emotional equilibrium; developing healthy coping strategies, recreational activities
8. Vocational rehabilitation	Assessment and training for vocational activities, assessment of further education needs or job modification
9. Follow-up	Lifelong prosthetic, functional, and medical assessment; emotional support

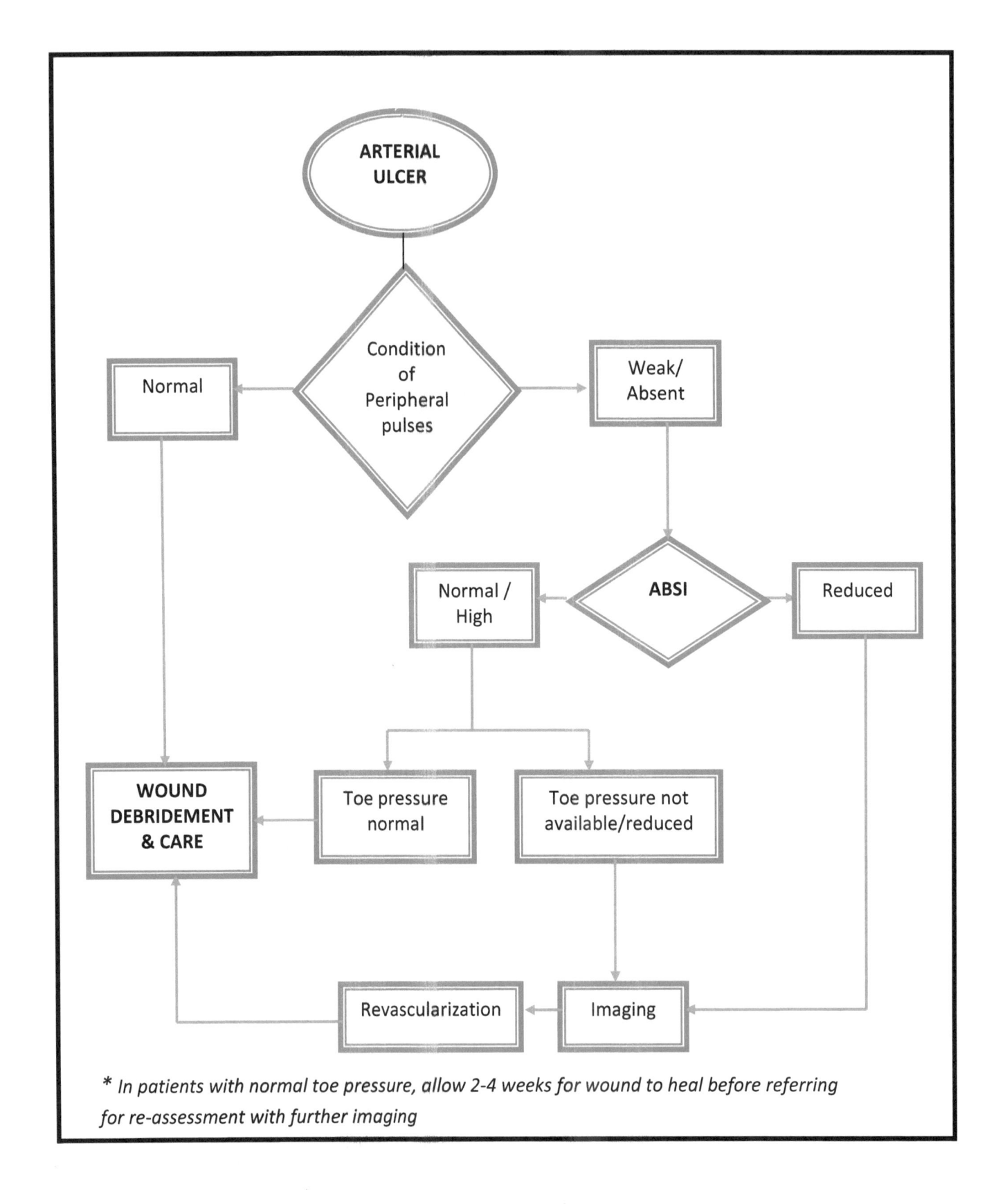

```
                    ┌─────────────┐
                    │  ARTERIAL   │
                    │   ULCER     │
                    └──────┬──────┘
                           │
                      ╱ Condition ╲
          ┌─────────╱      of       ╲─────────┐
          │ Normal ╲   Peripheral   ╱ Weak/Absent
          └────┬───╱     pulses    ╲───┬──────┘
               │        ╲       ╱      │
               │                       │
               │                    ╱ ABSI ╲
               │         ┌─────────╱        ╲─────────┐
               │         │ Normal/High      Reduced   │
               │         └──┬──────┬──────────────────┤
               │            │      │                  │
               │    Toe pressure   Toe pressure not   │
               │       normal      available/reduced  │
               │            │              │          │
               ▼            ▼              ▼          │
          ┌──────────────────────┐    ┌─────────┐     │
          │ WOUND DEBRIDEMENT    │◄───│ Imaging │◄────┘
          │      & CARE          │    └─────────┘
          └──────────────────────┘         │
                    ▲                      ▼
                    │              ┌──────────────────┐
                    └──────────────│ Revascularization│
                                   └──────────────────┘
```

* In patients with normal toe pressure, allow 2-4 weeks for wound to heal before referring for re-assessment with further imaging

Figure 8c.2 Algorithm for management of arterial ulcer

Conclusion

It is crucial to identify an arterial (ischaemic) ulcer, as the management of such an ulcer is different. Prompt intervention to improve the blood supply to the affected limb is important for healing of an ischemic ulcer.

Points to remember:
- Arterial ulcer is a reflection of a systemic disease. Care should be taken to assess the cardiovascular system.
- It is crucial to check for the peripheral pulses in all legs with ulcers. Absent pulses will require further assessment to exclude ischaemic ulcer
- Once identified, patients with ischaemic ulcers will require vascular intervention or revascularization
- Leg elevation and compression bandages must be avoided in all cases of suspected ischemic ulcers
- Pain management – ischaemic ulcer is extremely painful

References

1. *Inter-Society Consensus for the Management of Peripheral Arterial Disease (TASC II) European Journal Vascular and Endovascular SurgeryVol 33, Supplement 1, 2007*

2. *Hiatt WR. Medical Treatment of peripheral arterial disease and claudication. N Eng J Med. 2001;344:1608–21*

3. *J Am Podiatr Med Assoc 91(1): 13-22,2001) Alberto Esquenazi, MD,RobertDiGiacomo, PT*

Chapter 8: Management of Chronic Wound
d) Pressure Ulcer

Dr Khairiah Mohd Yatim/ Dr Zairizam Zakaria

8d-1. Definition

A pressure ulcer is localized injury to the skin and/or underlying tissue usually over a bony prominence, as a result of pressure, or pressure in combination with shear and/or friction. A number of contributing or confounding factors are also associated with pressure ulcers; the significance of these factors is yet to be elucidated. (NPUAP 2007)

8d-2. Pathophysiology

I) Primary Factors
- Pressure

    Kosiak 1961 Arch Phys Meds & Rehab (Animal Study)
    – There is an inverse relationship of pressure and time whereby,
    – Intense pressure, short duration, can be as damaging as lower intensity pressure for longer periods. furthermore Tissues can tolerates much higher cyclic pressure than constant pressure

- Shear
    – Occurs when skin remain static and underlying tissue shifts
    – Accounts for the high incident of sacral ulcer and when head of the bed is elevated more than 30 degree and less than 80 degree

- Friction
    – Occurs when skin moves against a support surface
    – Produces skin tear and abrasion

FRICTION + SHEAR + PRESSURE = EXTENSIVE INJURY

Refer Figure 8d.1 and Figure 8d.2 for the amount of pressure exerted on lying and sitting

II) Secondary Factors
- Elderly
- Limited mobility and prolonged bed rest.
- Decreased skin sensation.
- Moisture from bladder or bowel accidents
- Spasticity or improper transfer of patients in and out of chairs or beds can result in skin shearing and or friction

Figure 8d.1 Pressures exerted over bony prominences in supine and prone positions

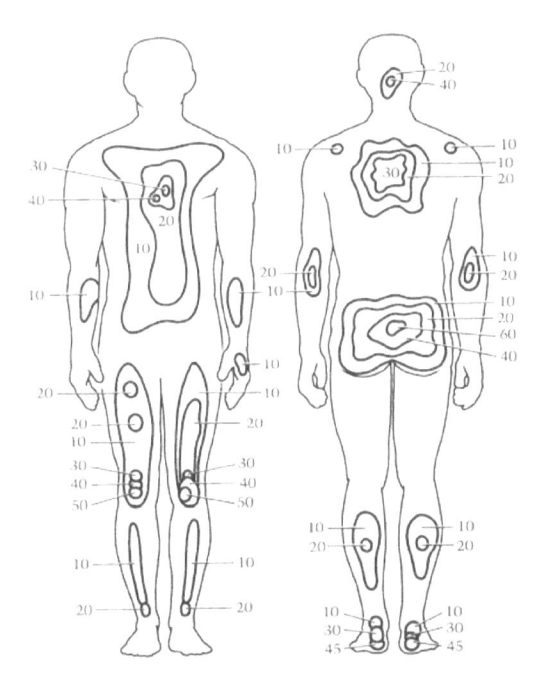

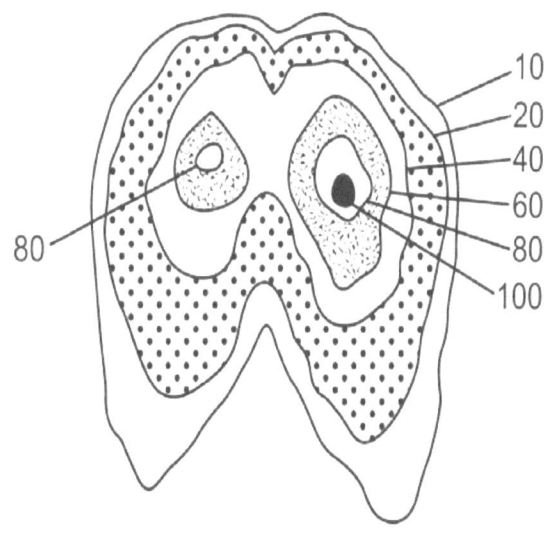

Figure 8d.2 Pressure exerted over bony prominences in sitting position.

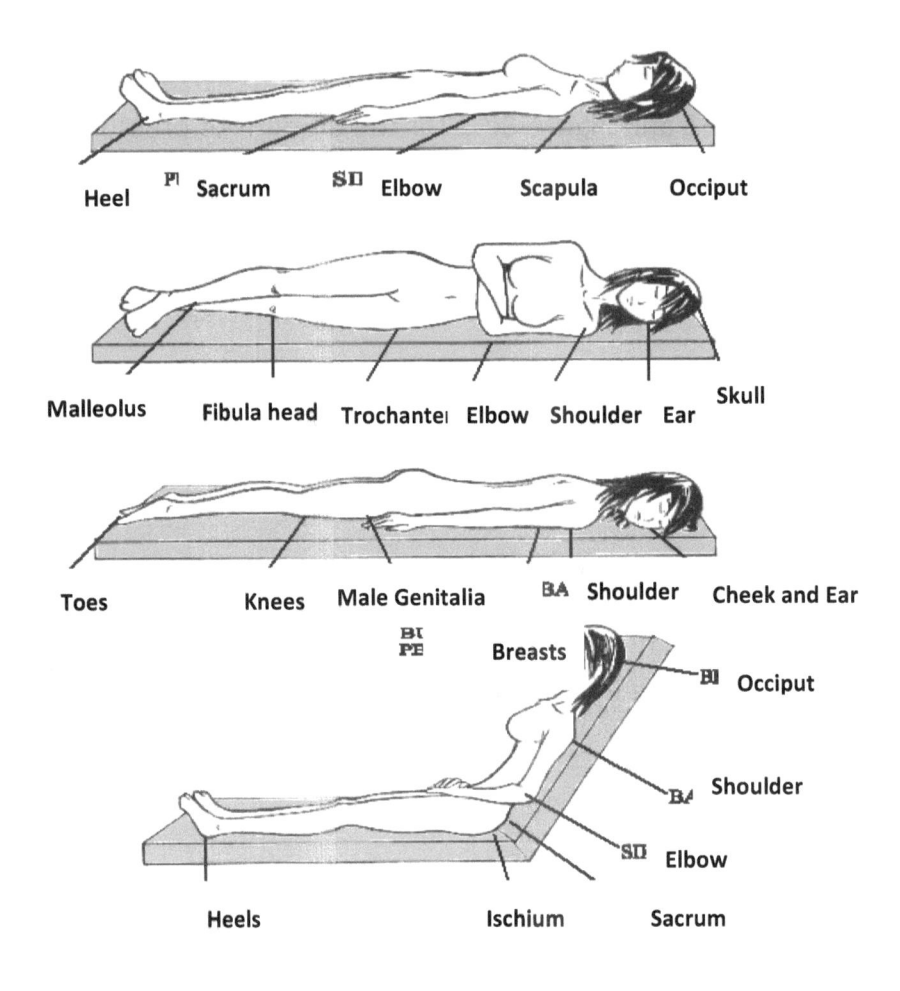

Figure 8d.3 Common Sites of Pressure Ulcers

- Associated co-morbidities such as Diabetes Mellitus, end-stage renal failures, anemia, small vessel occlusion disease, hypoproteinemia

- Poor nutritional status

- Poor psychosocial support

III) Clinical presentation

- Common sites for pressure ulcer to occur (Figure 8d.3)

IV) How to assess pressure ulcer

- Risk factor evaluation

    – To aid in the planning of appropriate preventive interventions, Barbara Braden and Nancy Bergstrom introduced a risk assessment scale (Braden scale) which is widely used in clinical setting (Appendix 4)

- Staging of pressure ulcer: Data from National Pressure Ulcer Advisory Panel (NPUAP); Table 8d-1.

- T.I.M.E. principle can be used as a guide to assess pressure ulcer and planning for its treatment

8d-3. Management

What is the best management of pressure ulcer?

1. Prevention is paramount

- Prevention is the main modality in the management of pressure ulcer.
- Proper bed positioning and turns every 2 hours (Figure 8d.4 and figure 8d.5)
- Bony prominence should be checked once or twice a day by the care giver.
- To provide the appropriate type of mattress-overlay or chair cushion to reduce pressure during sitting or lying.
- Best managed by a dedicated, multi-disciplinary team who has special interest in wound management.

2. **General treatment**

    - Restoration of tissue perfusion by relief of pressure
    - Treatment of underlying systemic problem e.g Anemia, Hypoprotenemia, Diabetes Mellitus
    - Treatment of reflex spasms- e.g. Baclofen, Diazepam and Tizanidine
    - Preventing or treating infection (refer national antibiotic guidelines)
    - Improvement in general health and nutrition.

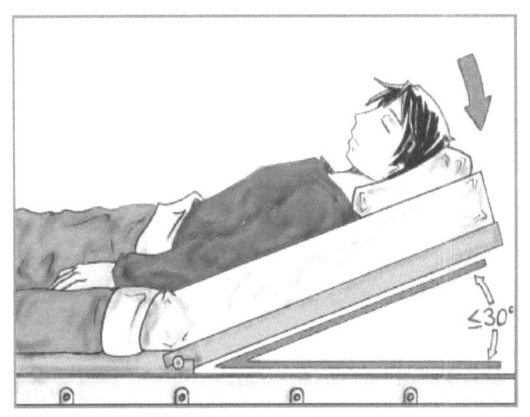

Figure 8d.4 Make sure the head end of the bed is propped up to not more than 30 degrees

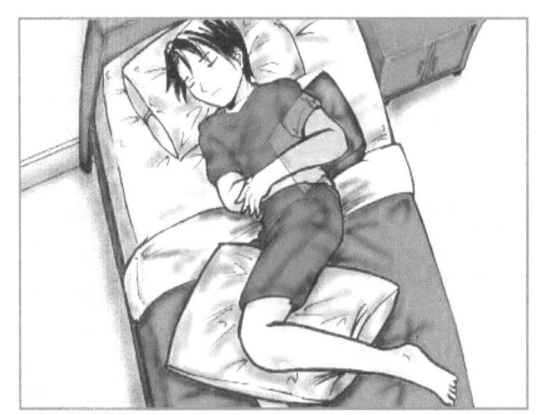

Figure 8d.5 Always provide appropriate padding to the pressure areas

Table 8d.1 Staging of Pressure Ulcer

Stage I: Intact skin with non-blanchable redness of a localized area usually over a bony prominence. Darkly pigmented skin may not have visible blanching; its color may differ from the surrounding area.	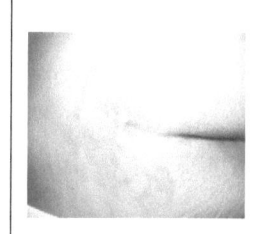
Stage II: Partial thickness loss of dermis presenting as a shallow open ulcer with a red pink wound bed, without slough. May also present as an intact or open/ruptured serum-filled blister.	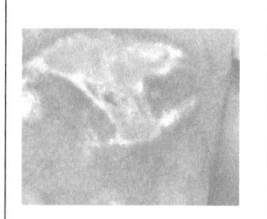
Stage III: Full thickness tissue loss. Subcutaneous fat may be visible but bone, tendon or muscle is not exposed. Slough may be present but does not obscure the depth of tissue loss. May include undermining and tunneling.	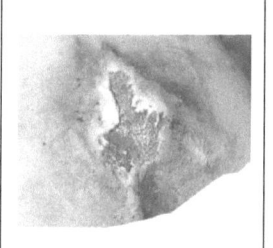
Stage IV: Full thickness tissue loss with exposed bone, tendon or muscle. Slough or eschar may be present on some parts of the wound bed. Often include undermining and tunneling.	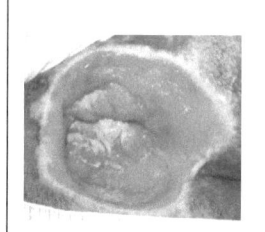
Unstageable: Full thickness tissue loss in which the base of the ulcer is covered by slough (yellow, tan, gray, green or brown) and/or eschar (tan, brown or black) in the wound bed.	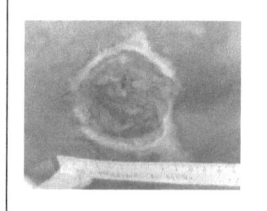

Suspected Deep Tissue Injury:
Purple or maroon localized area of discolored intact skin or blood-filled blister due to damage of underlying soft tissue from pressure and/or shear. The area may be preceded by tissue that is painful, firm, mushy, boggy, warmer or cooler as compared to adjacent tissue.

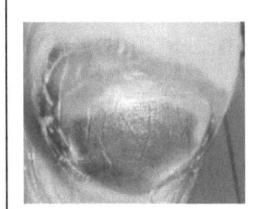

- Optimization of functional status and improving quality of life - role for Rehabilitation Physician, Occupational Therapist and Physiotherapist
- Cooperation with other services -role of psychologist, psychiatrist, social service worker
- Prevention of new ulcer development/recurrence

3. **Local treatment**
   - **Conservative:** Management of wounds - please refer algorithm on wound care
   - **Surgical:** Please refer chapter on principle of wound closure and wound debridement

---

Points to remember:

- Prevention is the most important in pressure ulcer management
- Small skin lesion may hide a large underlying wounds
- Management requires multidiscipline approach and family support
- Not all pressure ulcer patients are suitable for surgical intervention

References

1. *Plastic Surgery Second Edition (Mathes), 2006, Volume VI, Pg 1317-1353*

2. *Salcido R.,Goldman R., Prevention and Management of Pressure Ulcers and Other Chronic Wounds,:645-661 Phys. Med. &Rehab.,2nd ed. Braddom RL.*

3. *http://www.npuap.org/resources/educational-and-clinical-resources/npuap-pressure-ulcer-stagescategories/*

4. *BergstromN,BradenBJ,LaguzzaA,HolmanV.The Braden Scale for predicting pressure sore risk. Nurs Res. 1987;36(4):205-210.*

5. *KatrinBalzer, Claudia Pohl, Theo Dassen, Rudd Halfens: The Norton, Waterlow, Braden, and Care Dependency Scales Comparing Their Validity When Identifying Patients' Pressure Sore Risk. Journal of Wound, Ostomy and Continence Nursing:2007;34(4):389-398.*

6. *Linden, O., Greenway, R. M., and Piazza, J. M. Pressure distribution on the surface of the human body. I. Evaluation in lying and sitting positions using a "bed of springs and nails". Arch. Phys. Med. Rehabil. 46: 378, 1965.*

7. *Enis J, Sarmiento A: The pathophysiology and management of pressure sores. Othop Rev 2:26, 1973*

8. *Maklebust J: Pressure ulcers: etiology and prevention. NursClin North Am 22:359, 1987*

9. *Special thanks to Mohd. Asrul b. Mohd Noh . Illustrator*

CHAPTER 9
Management of Non-Healing Ulcer

Dr Andre Das

9-1. Definition

Any wound that has no signs of healing process within 2-4weeks after intervention by proper wound management team.

Features of non-healing wound:
- Size remain the same

- Persistent discharge

Arbitrary guide only (use personal clinical judgement to decide)

9-2. Causes

Usually multifactorial but can be broadly classified into the following factors

1. *Patient/Systemic:*
    - Malnutrition
    - Poorly controlled comorbid conditions e.g Diabetes
    - Smoking
    - Hygiene
    - Medication e.g Steroids/Chemotherapy
    - Pressure wounds
    - Patient immobility factors e.g. paraplegia
    - Appliance related e.g. poor fitting shoes

2. *Disease/Local:*
    - Arterial
    - Venous
    - Mixed Arterial and Venous
    - Infective e.g.
        1) +/- Biofilms
        2) Osteomyelitis
        3) Chronic infections e.g. TB/Fungal
    - Immunopathic including Pyoderma Gangrenosum
    - Malignancy
    - Post radiation
    - Systemic disease e.g. Connective Tissue Disease
    - Idiopathic

9-3. Management

Goals of Management

- Timely healing of wounds with minimal morbidity and best cosmetic and functional outcome
- Prevent recurrences
- Improve Quality of Life

Principles of Management

- Multidisciplinary Approach
- Careful Documentation of Progress of the Wound
- Utilisation of appropriate adjuncts where applicable

- Identify the cause if possible and treat
- Treat associated symptoms e.g. pain
- Consider Lifestyle Modifications
- Risk factor reduction to prevent recurrences

Clinical Assessment

History

Main Points:

- Duration of wound
- Symptoms caused by wounds
- Disability caused by wound
- Co-morbid history
- Medications
- Previous treatment
- Lifestyle
- Occupation

Examination

Color, Odor, Texture and Warmth are signs of infection

1. Inspection
    - Anatomical location especially whether over the lower limbs
    - Clues from the ulcer to suggest cause eg punched edges suggest arterial, rolled edges suggest malignancy
    - Area of ulcer
    - Cleanliness and associated unhealthy tissues

- Associated signs of disease eg trophic nail changes
- Suspicions of Pathergy (an immunopathic condition which is treated by immunosuppression) e.g violeceous edges

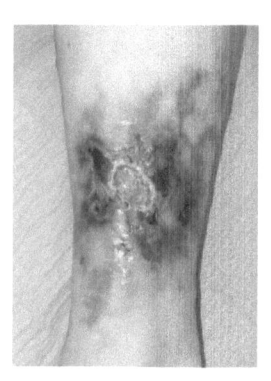

Picture of violeceous edges

Courtesy of Hardin Md Universiti of Iowa

2. Palpation
    - Tenderness to suggest associated infection
    - Neurovascular status
    - Tendons and movement

Investigations
    - X-ray for suspected bony involvement
    - Duplex for suspected vascular
    - Biopsy for suspected malignancy or chronic infection
    - Deep tissue cultures for suspected infections

9-4. Treatment

Toilet and debridement of Unhealthy Tissues and/or Biofilm:

- Surgical
- Hydrotherapy
- Enzymatic/Chemical
- Biological

Dressing

- Special wounds may require special dressing e.g. compression bandaging (refer to chapter on respective ulcer)
- Choice depends on local situation and resources
- Dressing is targeted to the current wound condition e.g. exudative requires absorbent dressings

9-5. Precautions

- Arterial ulcers are systemic disease which need to be looked into especially the cardiovascular state
- Malignancy may be secondary to the chronic ulcer i.e. Marjolin's ulcer
- Note any contraindications in specific treatment e.g.
    i. Graduated Compression Stockings cannot be used for arterial disease
    ii. Debridement of pathergic wounds

9-6. Adjuncts

1. Antibiotics:

    - Choice depends on disease, site, suspected pathogens and local sensitivity patterns.

    - Duration depends on similar reasons and the response pattern.

    - Ideally obtain deep tissue cultures before stating antibiotics.

    - Routine swab culture is generally discouraged.

    - Consider empirical antibiotics in the following situations

        i. Local conditions eg thickened skins in lipodermatosclerosis make it difficult to diagnose infections

        ii. Immunocompromised patients who may not show signs or symptoms of sepsis

2. Analgesics

3. Pentoxifylline for special ischemic ulcers

4. Off load devices for pressure associated ulcers

5. Stop Smoking

6. Splints: for immobilisation in special situations

7. Colostomy for certain perineal wounds

8. Continuos Bladder Drainage (CBD) for certain situations

9. Hyperbaric chamber if available for indicated wounds

9-7. Palliative Care

In the event the wound cannot be healed for whatever reason, consider palliative care

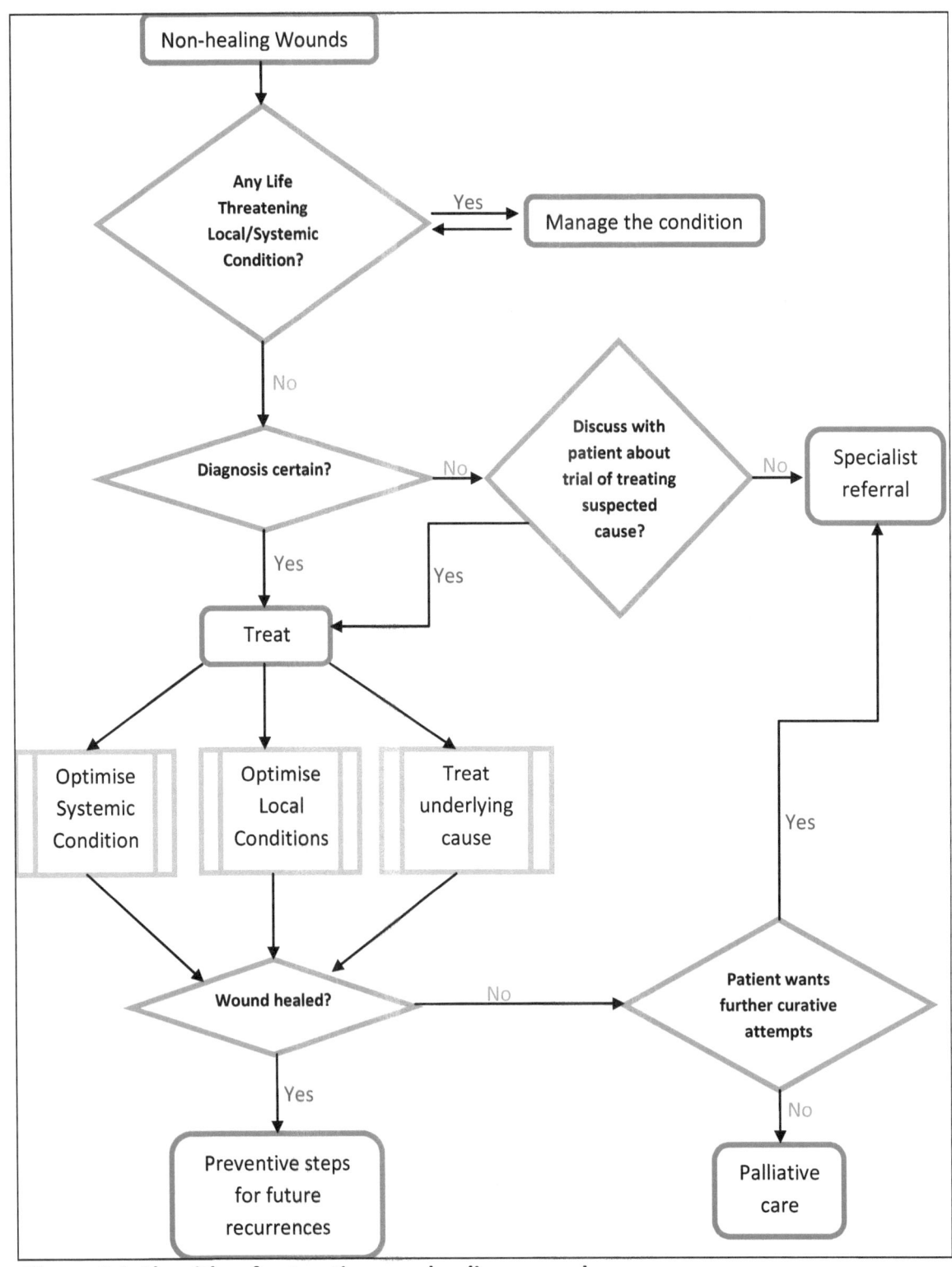

Figure 9.1 Algorithm for treating non-healing wounds

> **Point to Remember:**
> - You should recognize when a wound can be termed non-healing and may need specialised intervention.
>
> - Palliative care may be appropriate in certain situations. The possibility of malignant change in such ulcers must also be remembered.

References

1. *ABC of arterial and venous disease: ulcerated lower limb BMJ volume 320 10JUNE2000*

2. *The Non Healing Wound(Review) MMW Fortschr Med. 2004 Oct 28;146(44):45-8.(Translated from German)*

3. *Care of chronic wounds in palliative care and end-of-life patients Int Wound J. 2010 Aug;7(4):214-35.*

4. *Complex Wounds Clinics (Sao Paulo). 2006 Dec;61(6):571-8.*

5. *Diagnosis and treatment of pyoderma gangrenosum BMJ VOLUME 333 22 JULY 2006*

6. *Outcomes in controlled and comparative studies on nonhealing wounds: recommendations to improve the quality of evidence in wound management. Journal of Wound Care Vol 19 No 6 June 2010*

CHAPTER 10: Management of Life-Threatening Wounds

Dr Mohammad Anwar Hau Abdullah

10-1. Introduction

Necrotizing fasciitis (NF):

- Necrotizing fasciitis is potentially fatal infection characterized by rapid progression with widespread necrosis of the subcutaneous tissue and superficial fascia. The infection may also leads to gas production and sepsis. It is more likely to occur in immune compromised people.

- Subtype of NF and the causative organism:

Subtype	Bacteriology	Known as
Type I	Polymicrobial	
Type II	Group A beta hemolytic *Streptococcal* (*Streptococcus pyogenes*), *Staphylococcus aureus*	Flash eating bacteria
Type III	-*Clostridium perfringens*, *C. novyi* *Bacteroides fragilis*.	Gas gangrene

10-2. Incidence

Necrotising fasciitis

- Absolute data for the incidence and prevalence of necrotising fasciitis is not known. But it is known that Type I is more common than Type II necrotising fascitis.

10-3. Pathophysiology

Necrotising fasciitis

- Bacteria are introduced into the skin through a decrease in tissue resistance often as a result of immunosuppression.

- Infection spread along the subcutaneous tissue, and fascia aided by the release of bacterial toxins and enzymes; such as hyaluronidase, collagenase, streptokinase, and lipase.

- Uninhibited progression of bacterial penetration results in tissue necrosis and thrombosis of the vasculature.

Type III NF (gas gangrene):

- The infection is usually due to direct inoculation and with the present of anaerobic environment, the bacteria produce toxins that cause muscle death, lead to shock and red blood cell destruction (haemolysis)

- Progression to toxemia and shock is often very rapid, and may cause death within 24 hours

10-4. Clinical presentation

Necrotising fasciitis:

- Early presentation: erythema (redness), pain, and edema in the affected limb
- The infection- rapid spreading of erythema, ecchymosis with vesicles enlarging to purple bullae; inside these purple bullae is a foul smelling, thin, watery fluid known as "dishwater pus"; the bullae may be hemorrhagic.
- Crepitus may be felt (especially in patient with gas gangrene).
- The patient is normally very sick and toxic appearance.

10-5. Assessment

General:

- Vital signs
- Signs of sepsis
- Pain score
- Hydration status, urine output, hemoglobin level, arterial blood gases
- Co-morbid illness

Local:

- NF is clinical diagnosis which has to be recognized and diagnose early.
- The affected leg is swollen with erythema, warm and tender (rule out DVT)
- Haemorrhagic bullae and crepitus may be present.
- The infection can spread very rapidly.

Investigations:

- Blood count, ESR, CRP
- EGC, Chest x-ray and other relevant investigations.
- Plain x-ray of the affected foot/leg: soft tissue swelling and presence of air.
- Ultrasound: to rule out DVT; demonstrate fluid/edema in the soft tissue.

10-6. Management

Fundamental to the successful treatment of necrotising fasciitis (and gas gangrene) is early diagnosis, early administration of appropriate antibiotics, and rapid surgical debridement.

General

- Early systemic broad-spectrum antibiotics which must cover the most likely organisms. The antibiotic is then switched according to the tissue bacteriology report.

- Other general supportive managements depending on the patients' presentation and condition.

Local

- Aggressive wide, extensive surgical excision and drainage to remove all infected, necrotic tissue and fascia or muscles until clean, healthy, pearly gray fascia or muscles is identified in all margins of the wound should be performed as soon as the diagnosis of necrotizing fasciitis or gas gangrene is made to arrest the infection process.

- Do not hesitate to perform repeated debridement if clinically indicated or even in doubt.

- In small percentage of patient amputation may be necessary or indicated in order to save life.

- If available, hyperbaric oxygen therapy may be used as adjuvant treatment.

- Post-debridement; the general management of the wound follows the flow chart in "Chapter 17: Algorithm for Wound Care Treatment".

10-7. Clinical photos

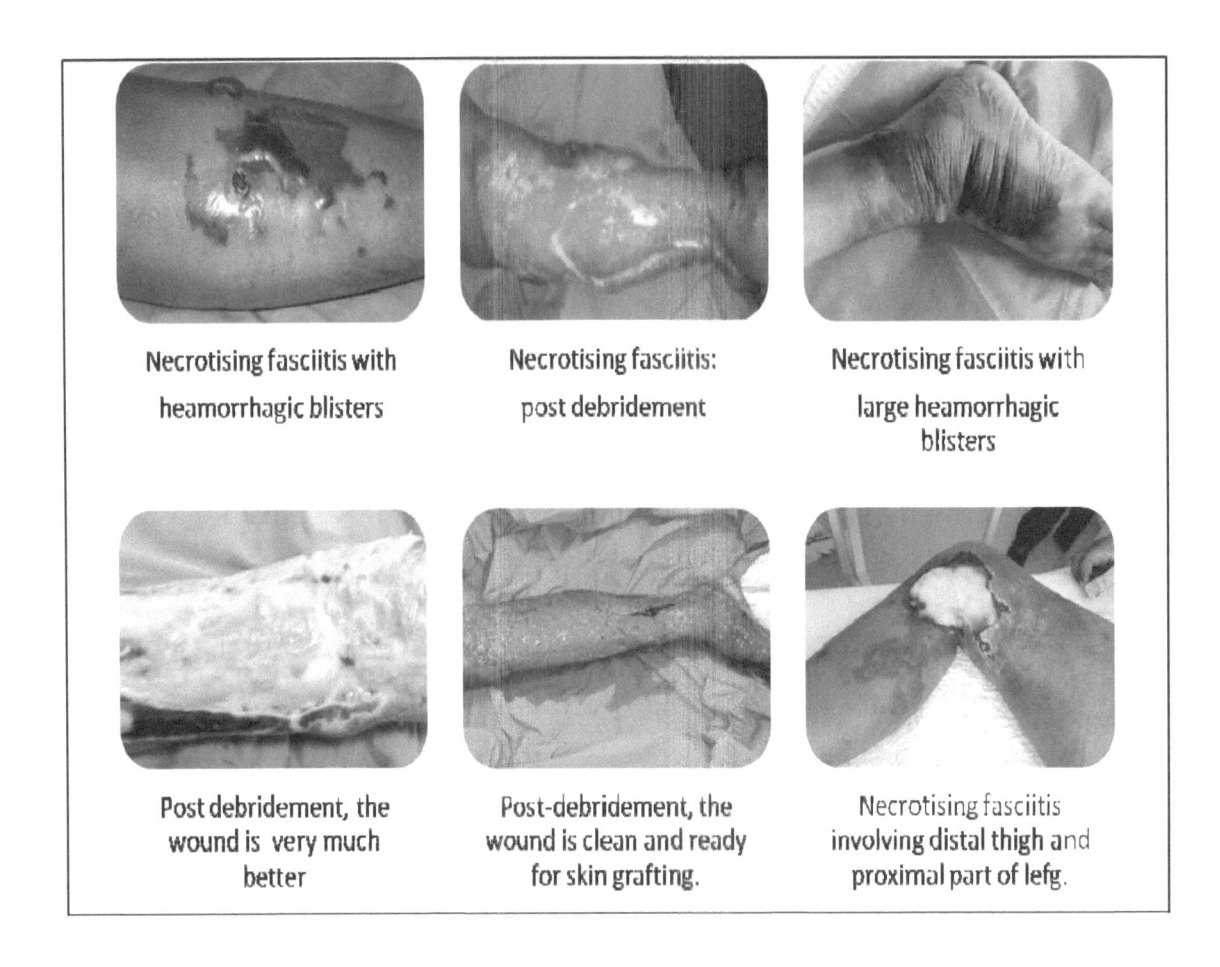

Figure 10.1 Clinical photos of necrotizing fasciitis

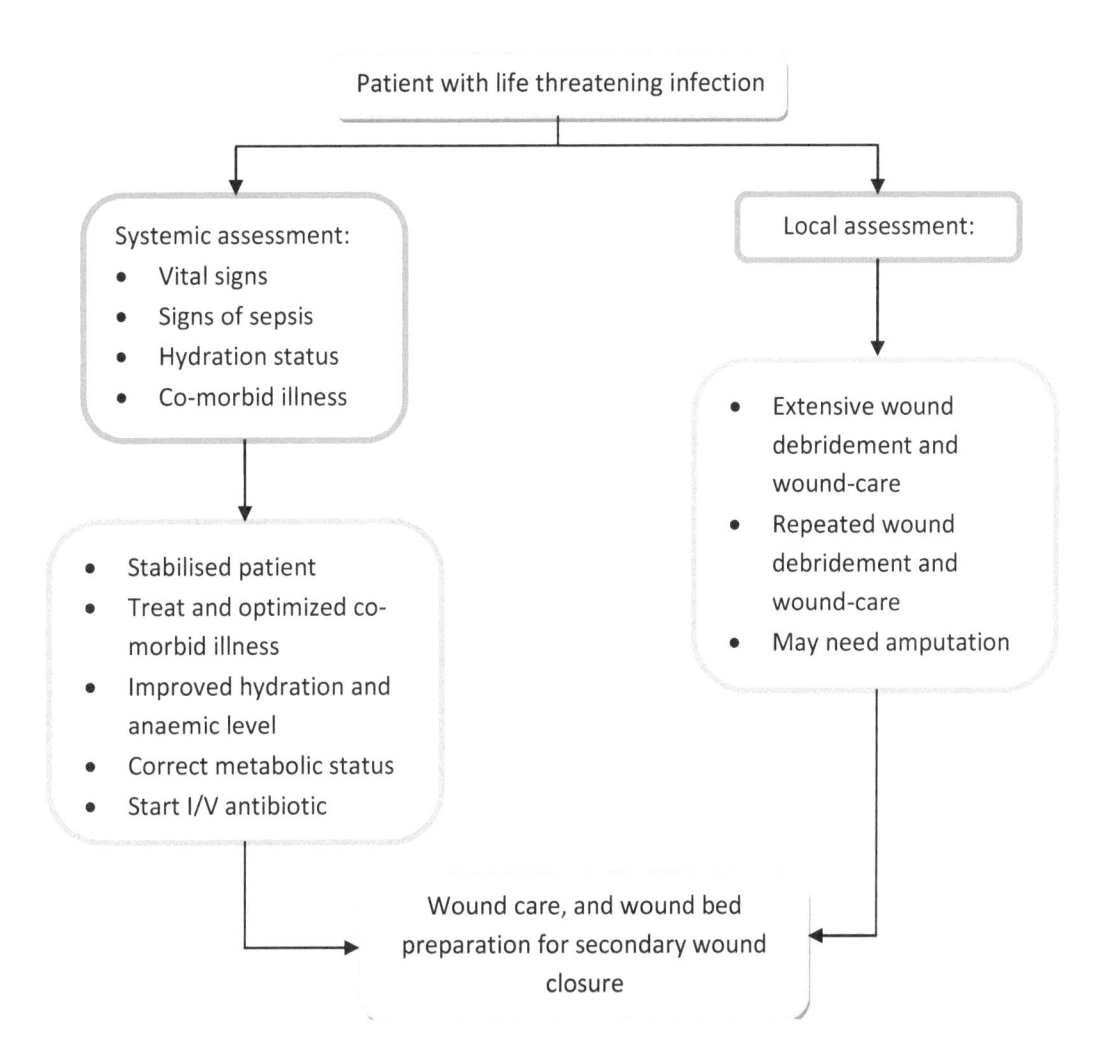

```
Patient with life threatening infection
                │
        ┌───────┴───────┐
        ▼               ▼
Systemic assessment:          Local assessment:
• Vital signs                       │
• Signs of sepsis                   ▼
• Hydration status            • Extensive wound
• Co-morbid illness             debridement and
        │                       wound-care
        ▼                     • Repeated wound
• Stabilised patient            debridement and
• Treat and optimized co-       wound-care
  morbid illness             • May need amputation
• Improved hydration and
  anaemic level
• Correct metabolic status
• Start I/V antibiotic
        │                           │
        └──────────┬────────────────┘
                   ▼
        Wound care, and wound bed
        preparation for secondary wound
        closure
```

Figure 10.2 Flow chart in management of life-threatening wound

> Point to Remember:
> - Necrotising fasciitis is a potentially life threatening infection.
> - Early diagnosis and prompt treatment is the most crucial for patient's prognosis

References

1. Das DK, Baker MG, Venugopal K. Increasing incidence of necrotizing fasciitis in New Zealand: A nationwide study over the period 1990 to 2006. J Infect. 2011 Dec;63(6):429-33.

2. Edlich RF et. Al. Modern concepts of the diagnosis and treatment of necrotizing fasciitis. J Emerg Med. 2010 Aug; 39(2):261-5.

3. Naqvi GA, Malik SA, Jan W. Necrotizing fasciitis of the lower extremity: a case report and current concept of diagnosis and management. d J Trauma Resusc Emerg Med. 2009 Jun 15;17:28

4. Maynor ME. Emergent Management of Necrotizing Fasciitis. Medscape. June 2011.

5. Shukla A. Gas Gangrene in Emergency Medicine. Medscape. June 2011.

CHAPTER 11: Analgesia for Wound Dressing Related Procedures

Dr Kavita Bhojwani/ Dr Mary Cardosa/ Dr Harijah Wahidin

11-1. Introduction

'Pain is an important aspect of wound care. "Unresolved pain negatively affects wound healing and has an impact on the quality of life. Pain at wound dressing procedures can be managed by a combination of accurate assessment, suitable dressing choices, skilled wound management and individualized analgesic regimens. For therapeutic as well as humanitarian reasons, it is vital that clinicians know how to assess, evaluate and manage pain (ref 2)'

11-2. Types of pain

1. Background pain

- The pain felt at rest, when no wound manipulation is taking place.
- May be continuous (e.g. like a toothache) or intermittent (e.g. like cramp or night-time pain).
- Related to the underlying cause of the wound, local wound factors (e.g. ischemia, infection and maceration) and other related pathologies (e.g. diabetic neuropathy, peripheral vascular disease, rheumatoid arthritis and dermatological conditions).

2. Incident (breakthrough) pain

- The pain that may occur during day-to-day activities (e.g. mobilisation, coughing, repositioning).

3. Procedural pain

- Results from a procedure such as dressing change and simple wound debridement

11-3. Assessment of Pain

Assessment of pain is essential for accurate management.

1. *Ask the patient about his/her pain*

    - At regular intervals, whenever the BP/P/RR/Temp (vital signs) are taken (Pain as the 5th Vital sign).
    - Before, during and after dressing change.
    - Before, during and after a procedure (e.g. debridement).
    - At any other time when the patient complains of pain.

2. *When asking the patient about pain, record the Pain Score using any of the following pain scales (Appendix 5)*
    - Visual Analogue Scale / Numerical Rating Scale for adults and older children

    - Wong-Baker Faces Scale for children aged 1-4 years

3. *The analgesic administered should follow the pain score* (Appendix 5) (mild = pain score 1-3, moderate = pain score 4-6, severe = pain score more than 6)

11-4. Management

1. Background Pain

Non-pharmacological management
- a. Splinting
- b. Immobilization
- c. Relaxation / imagery

Pharmacological management

Analgesics are given according to the severity (pain score) of pain. (Refer analgesic ladder in Appendix 6 and List of Drugs used as analgesics in Appendix 7)

- a. Regular (6 - 8 hourly) Oral Paracetamol

(+/-)

- b. Regular NSAIDS or COX2 inhibitors (dosage depends on the drug);
  - Caution in patients with thrombocytopenia, coagulopathies, asthma and renal, hepatic or cardiac impairment.
  - Contraindicated for patients with hypovolemia, active peptic ulceration or with a history of sensitivity to aspirin or other NSAIDS.

(+/-)

- c. Regular (6 - 8 hourly) Weak opioids (Dihydrocodeine (DF118) or Tramadol)
  - Dosage to follow the analgesic ladder, depending on the level of pain (mild, moderate or severe)

❖ In patients who are unable to take orally, the above drugs may be replaced by any of the following
  - Regular (6 - 8 hourly) Rectal Paracetamol
  - Regular (8 hourly) Rectal Diclofenac
  - COX2 inhibitor – IV Parecoxib (but can only be given for maximum of 2 days)
  - Regular Subcutaneous Morphine 2.5-5 mg (4 hourly) or Tramadol 50-100 mg (6hourly) (max dose for tramadol is 400mg in a day)

- ❖ For patients with severe pain refer to Acute Pain Service (APS) or anaesthesiologist if no APS available.

- ❖ As all analgesics are associated with adverse effects, it is important to be aware of the contraindications and potential adverse effects and to treat side effects (e.g. nausea/vomiting) when they occur.

2. Incident Pain

All patients must be allowed to have "PRN" doses of analgesics to cover incident pain.

The actual analgesic and the dose depend on the analgesia prescribed for the background pain.

However, if there is a lot of breakthrough pain present, it will be necessary to review the   background analgesics.

Non-pharmacological management

    a.   Adequate preparation of the patient

    b.   Relaxation / imagery

Pharmacological management
a. For patients not requiring any regular analgesics (i.e. background pain is none or mild), a. prescribe PRN Paracetamol or NSAID (e.g. diclofenac)

b. For patients on regular paracetamol and/or NSAIDs (max dose for diclofenac is 50 mg 3 doses) or COXIBs, prescribe PRN Tramadol 50 mg or DF118 30-60 mg

c. For patients on regular PCM plus NSAIDs/COXIBs plus weak opioid (Tramadol or DF118) - prescribe additional (PRN) dose of the weak opioid (maximum dose of tramadol is 400 mg / day and maximum dose of DF118 is 240 mg / day)

d. Patients requiring strong opioids (e.g. morphine) should be co-managed with the APS or anaesthesiologist.

3. Procedural Pain

    a. Non-pharmacological management:

- Adequate preparation of the patient
- Use of non-traumatic dressings
- Soaking dressings before removal
- Allowing patient control (e.g. allowing the patient to determine the time of the dressing)
- Relaxation / imagery

    b. Pharmacological management:

Most analgesics can be administered before a painful event. Analgesia may be continued post-procedure, but if wound pain persists and is poorly controlled, background medication should be reviewed

    i. Oral route

- Paracetamol and NSAIDs should be given at least 1 hour prior to the procedure. It can be given together with oral weak opioids like DF118 or Tramadol

- When pain is difficult to control, strong opioids like immediate release formulations of oxycodone (Oxynorm 5- 10mg 4hrly PRN) and aqueous morphine (2.5-5mg 4hrly PRN)

- May also be administered orally half an hour prior to the procedure

    ii. Subcutaneous route

Used for severe pain during the procedure, when the above oral analgesics are inadequate to control the pain.

S/C Morphine
- ➢ To be given at least 30 minutes before the procedure is performed
- ➢ Dose depends on age of patient and severity of pain

  e.g. < 65yrs : 5mg -10mg

    > 65yrs : 2.5mg -5mg

iii. Intravenous route

Caution: All the following should only be given by doctors who have been trained in the administration of the analgesic to be used.

IV morphine 0.5 -1 mg bolus

Analgesia may be achieved using the morphine pain protocol (appendix 9). This involves the administration of IV morphine 0.5 -1 mg bolus, repeated every 5 minutes, titrated to effect (i.e. a reduction in pain score) and monitoring for side effects (drowsiness and respiratory depression) using the respiratory rate and the sedation score. (Appendix 8). Monitoring of SpO2 can also be done if available. If PCA is available, IV PCA morphine with a bolus dose of 1-2 mg and a lockout interval of 5 minutes may be used during the procedure, with the advice of the Acute Pain Service anaesthetist

IV Fentanyl 0.5 mcg/kg

slow bolus to be given 5-10 minutes before the procedure, repeated during the procedure if necessary, up to a maximum of 2 mcg/kg (total dose), with the advice of the Acute Pain Service anaesthetist
If PCA is available, IV PCA fentanyl with a bolus dose of 10-20 mcg and a lockout interval of 2-3 minutes may be used during the procedure, with the advice of the Acute Pain Service anaesthetist

Note:
i) The difference between IV morphine and IV fentanyl is in the onset and duration of action, with IV fentanyl having a faster onset but shorter

duration of action. Fentanyl is also more potent than morphine and can rapidly cause profound sedation and respiratory depression.

ii) Before removing the dressing, assess the pain by pressing over the wound. If the patient gives a pain score of 3 or more, further analgesia is required.

IV Ketamine

- 0.25 - 0.5 mg/kg titrated to effect.
- Usually used in children, but may be used in adults in selected cases.
  Note that the patient may have hallucinations with the use of this drug and IV midazolam 1-2 mg may have to be used concomitantly

IV. Topical local anaesthethics

Lignocaine

- Lignocaine (2% in 5-10 mls of normal saline)
- Plain lignocaine max dose 3mg/kg body wt;
- Lignocaine with adrenaline max dose is 7mg/kg body wt
- Soaked gauze over the wound; allow to sit on the wound for 3-5 mins before procedure.
- Can provide a degree of numbness.

v. Inhalational

Methoxyflurane (Penthrox)
- Used as an inhaler 5 minutes prior to procedure
- Each inhaler can be used multiple times by the same patient
- The maximum dose of methoxyflurane via the inhaler is:
- 3mL to 6 mL for a single episode of severe pain
- 15mL in any 7 day period (5 x 3mL bottles)
- Can only be used once in 48 hours (alternate day administration)

- ❖ Contraindications
  - Severe renal impairment with reduced glomerular infiltration rate (GFR) <30 mL per minute
  - Renal failure
  - Hypersensitivity to fluorinated anaesthetics
  - Cardiovascular instability
  - A history of possible adverse reactions in either patient or relatives
  - Patients unable to hold the inhaler due to impaired consciousness/cooperation
  - Patients who are intoxicated with alcohol or illicit drugs
  - Patients with respiratory depression, airway obstruction or airway burns
  - Patients susceptible to or having a family history of Malignant Hyperthermia
  - Concurrent use of tetracycline and other antibiotics of known nephrotoxic potential are not recommended as it may result in fatal renal toxicity

- ❖ Precautions
  - Diabetic patients
  - Liver disease

Uncontrolled Pain

Patients whose pain is not controlled despite all the above methods should be referred to the Acute Pain team (APS). There are other methods including the use of regional blocks (e.g. epidural, peripheral nerve block) which can be used in selected cases but this can only be done with the appropriate expertise and monitoring.

Antiemetics

Nausea and vomiting are common side effect of opioids.

There is no need to stop the opioids but it is necessary to treat the nausea and vomiting with antiemetics.

- Metoclopramide (maxalon)
  10-20mg IV/SC/oral - give one dose stat and repeat if necessary 6-8hrly

  If the patient continues to vomit or have nausea, then use

- Odansetron 4mgIV – give one dose stat and repeat if necessary 8 hrly

OR

- Granisetron 1mg IV - give one dose stat and repeat if necessary 8 hrly

Patient Education

It is necessary to educate patients with regards to their analgesic usage.
They must understand that in the beginning for the first 3-7 days, they will require to take their analgesics on a regular basis and then as the wound heals, it can be on a PRN basis.

It should be emphasized that prior to any procedure that they may require, they will need to ingest their analgesic 1 hour before the procedure. This may mean they take the medication at home before arriving at the clinic.

References

1. *Ezike HA et al   Oral ketamine for wound care procedures in adult patients with burns South Africa J Anaesth Analg 2011;17(3): 242-248*

2. *Principles of Best Practice, A world union of wound healing Societies Initiative – Minimising pain of wound dressing related procedures. A concensus document*

3. *Sussman C et al Wound Care: a collaborative practical manual*

4. *J LatarjetMD.Consultant in Anaesthesiology and Intensive Care; Chief, Burn Centre St Joseph and St Luc Hospital Lyon, France -The management of pain associated with dressing changes in patients with burns*

5. *Choiniere M, Melzack R, Rondeau J, Girard N, Paquin MJ. The pain of burns: characteristics and correlates. J Trauma 1989; 29(11): 1531-9.*

6. *Choiniere M, Auger FA, Latarjet J. Visual analogue thermometer: a valid and useful instrument for measuring pain in burned patients. Burns 1994; 20(3): 229-35.*

7. *McGrath PG. Pain in Children. New York: Guildford Press, 1990.*

8. *Recommendations from the Prince of Wales Drug and Therapeutic Committee, Dec 2005*

9. *Grindlay, J., Franz Babl E.F., Review article: Efficacy and safety of methoxyflurane analgesia in the emergency department and prehospital setting. Emergency Medicine Australasia, 2009, 21: 4–11.*

10. *Cousins, M.J, Mazze R.I, Methoxyflurane Nephrotoxicity. A Study of Dose Response in Man. JAMA, 1973, Vol 225, 13: 1611-1616*

11. *Marshall, M. A, Ozoria, H.P.L, Analgesia for Burns Dressing using Methoxyflurane. British Journal of Anaesthesia, 1972, 44:80-82*

12. *Tomi, K., et al. Alterations in pain threshold and psychomotor response associated with subanaesthetic concentrations of inhalation anaesthetics in humans. British Journal of Anaesthesia, 1993; 70:684-686*

13. *Pain as the 5th Vital Sign, Guidelines for Doctors – Management of Adult Patients Ministry of Health, Malaysia*

SECTION C:
Practical Aspect in Wound Care

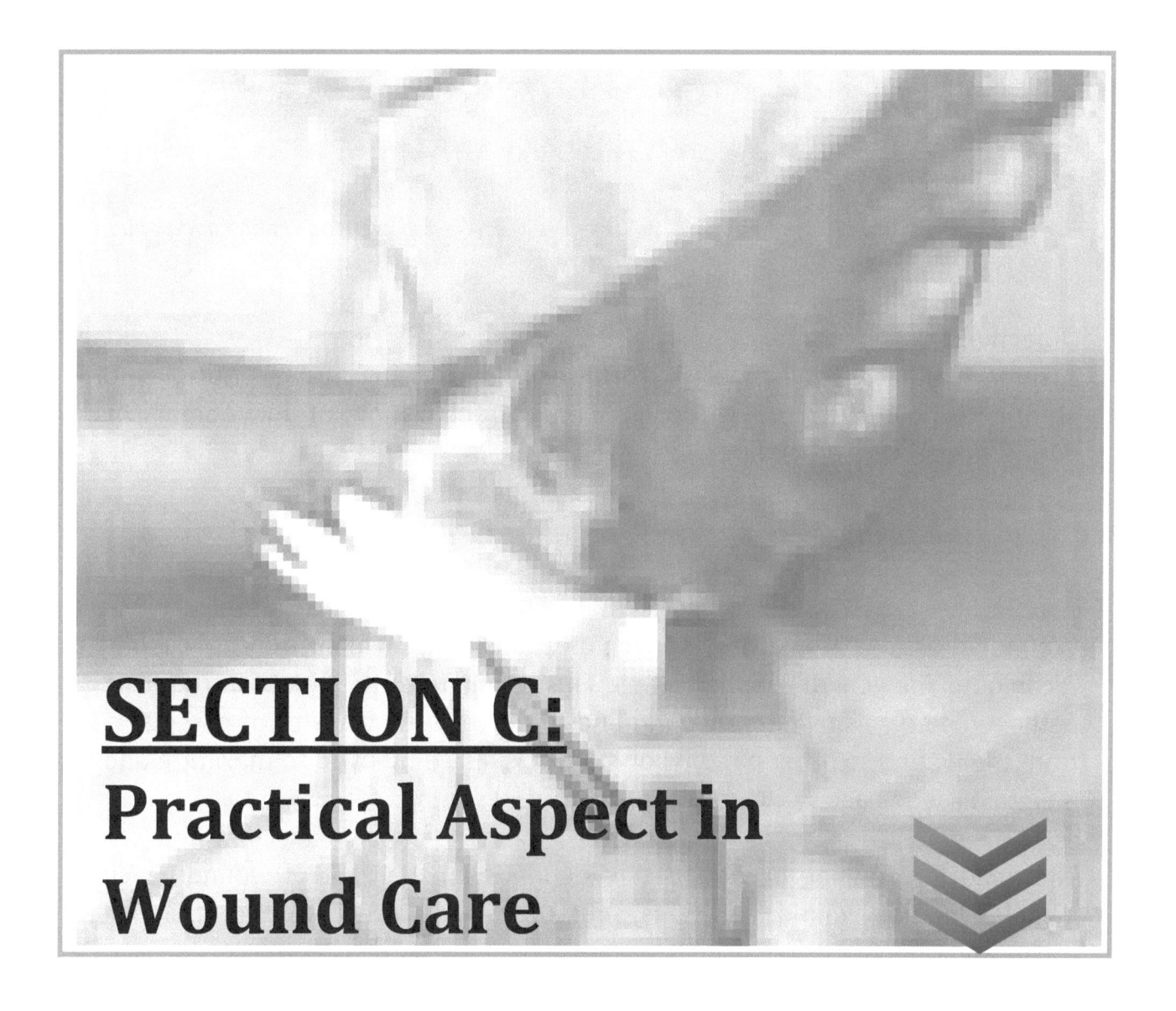

CHAPTER	TOPIC	CONTRIBUTORS
Chapter 12	Standard Operating Procedure on Wound Dressing	*Matron Leong*
Chapter 13	Wound Cleansing	*Dr Zairudin*
Chapter 14	Type of Dressing	*Dr Harikrishna*
Chapter 15	Wound Debridement	*Dr Mohamed Yusof* *Dr Zairudin* *Dr Harikrishna*

Chapter 16	Adjunctive Treatment
	   a) Honey Treatment
	   b) Hyperbaric Oxygen Therapy
	   c) Negative Pressure Wound Therapy (NPWT)
		Dr Mohamad Izani
		Dr Mohd Zamzuri/Dr Muhd Yusof
		Dr Normala

Chapter 17	Algorithm for Wound Care Treatment	*Dr Mohammad Anwar Hau*

CHAPTER 12
Standard Operating Procedure on Wound Dressing

Matron Leong Foong Khuan

Objectives:
Ensure healthcare personnel perform wound dressing using principles of aseptic technique to prevent or minimize transmission of microorganisms during wound care procedures.

12-1. Introduction

Wound dressing is a core nursing responsibility which utilizes aseptic technique. The goal of aseptic technique is to minimize the risk of introducing pathogenic organisms into a wound and to prevent the transfer of pathogens from the wound to other patients or staff. It is also employed to maximize and maintain asepsis and is applicable in any clinical setting.

The need for dressing or wound care depends on the type of wound which includes incision wound, abrasions, pressure ulcers, ulcers, wound at site of drains and others.

The attending health care personnel may require different wound technique for each type of wounds. However, the choice of wound dressing should be large enough to cover and protect the wound site and tissue around it. It should allow air circulation, safely secured to prevent slippage and is comfortable to patient.

STANDARD :

The nurses observe principles of medical asepsis during wound dressing to minimize introduction of potential infection and or its spread.

12-1. Wound Dressing Procedure

No	Process
1.	- Greet / acknowledge patient. - Provide privacy - Explain the procedure. - Identify type of wound dressing required. Infected or dirty wound dressing should be done last - Perform pain assessment - Administer analgesic if indicated.
2. 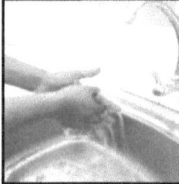 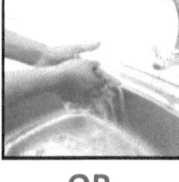 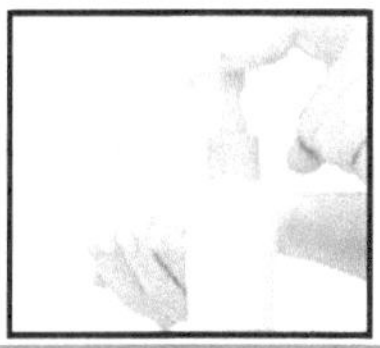	- Perform hand hygiene (observe 5 moments for hand hygiene) using soap and water OR alcohol based hand rub - Wear mask - Prepare trolley for dressing - Provide privacy - Place patient in a confortable position
3. 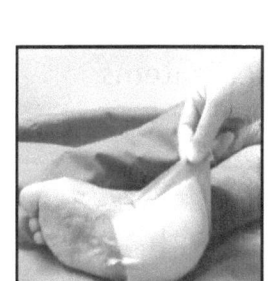	Loosen dressing: - Perform hand hygiene. Wear gloves (unsterile). - Loosen the existing dressing but do not remove it - Use saline or water for irrigation to further loosen the dressing if necessary - Remove gloves
4. 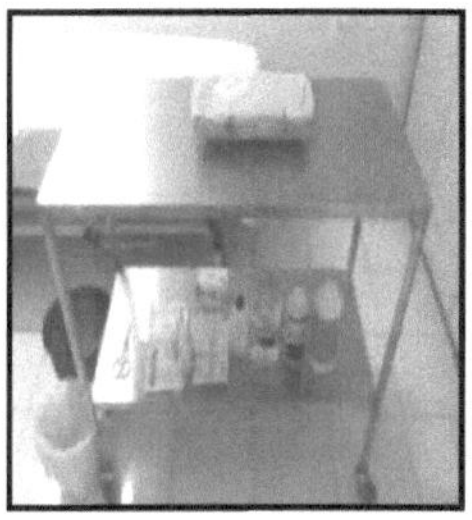	Perform Hand Hygiene. Prepare dressing requirements : - clean dressing trolley - sterile dressing set – top trolley - dressing materials- bottom trolley - cleansing solution– bottom trolley - Plaster/bandage, Scissor - clinical waste bin - General waste bin. - Check expiry date

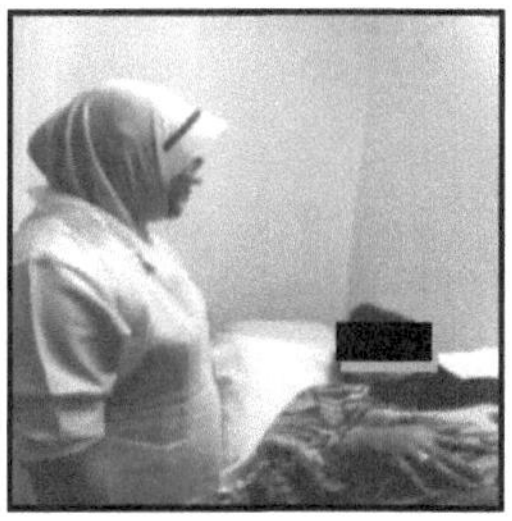

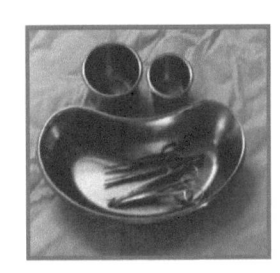

No		Process
5.		A complete dressing set should consists of: - kidney dish (1) - galipots (2) - Non-tooth dissecting forceps (2) - Bryant's dressing forceps (2)
6.		Perform hand hygiene. - Open dressing set. - Add the right quantity of sterile dressing materials. - Pour cleansing agent. - Maintain sterile field:- - Non sterile person should not reach across sterile areas or touch sterile item - Non sterile person should not contaminate sterile items when opening, disposing or transferring them to the sterile area - Place only sterile items within the sterile area - The sterile person should not reach across unsterile areas or touch unsterile items
7.		Perform hand hygiene. - Wear sterile gloves. - Remove loosen soiled dressing with a pair of forceps. - Discard used forceps into receiver (bottom trolley) - Perform wound assessment. Inform attending doctor if there is any concern.
8.		Prepare swabs for dressing - Dip swabs into cleansing solution and squeeze excessive cleansing solution.

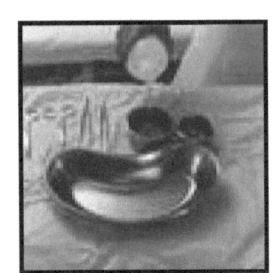

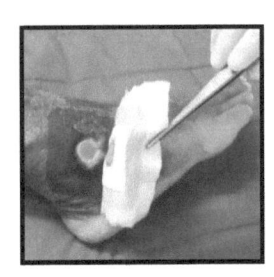

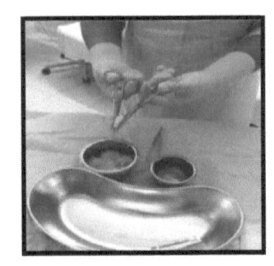

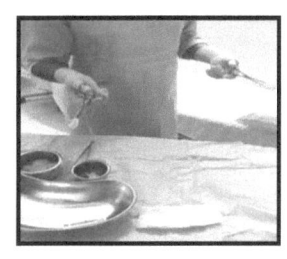

No	Process
9.	- Keep forceps facing downward and above waist line when performing dressing. - Avoid the soiled forceps (forceps in contact with the wound) from touching the sterile field.
10.	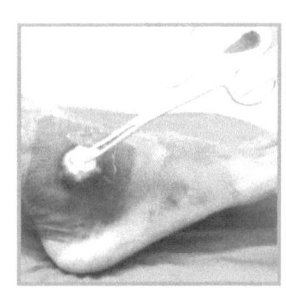 Perform dressing as according to the sequence below: - Swab from clean area to dirty area. Use one swab for each stroke. - Remove debris, scabs, slough, biofilm when necessary. - Irrigate with non antiseptic solution if required - Clean the peri-wound area thoroughly.
11.	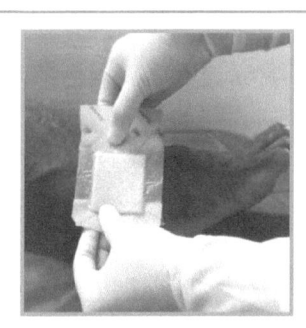 Choice of Dressings: - Apply non-allergenic dressing. To promote healing - Use of appropriate off-loading device if required. - Ensure the wound is completely covered with appropriate dressing. - Secure dressing appropriately so as not to impair blood circulation.
12.	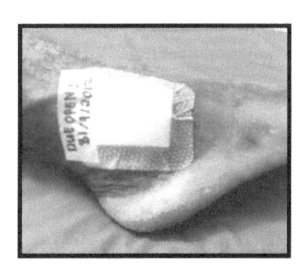 Label dressing done: - Date dressing done. - Date due for next dressing.
13.	- Clear trolley. Used dressing set to be sent to Central Sterile Supply Unit (CSSU) for re-sterilization - Perform hand hygiene.

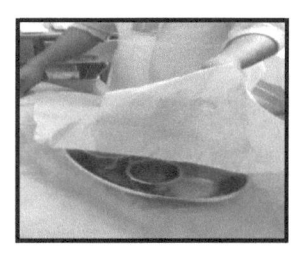

No	Process
14.	**Health Education** - Inform patient wound progress. - Maintain a well-balanced diet. - Compliance to medication and follow up treatment. - Personal hygiene.
15.	Document wound findings and care rendered in wound care chart.

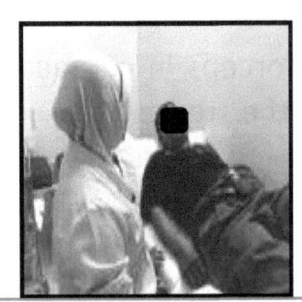

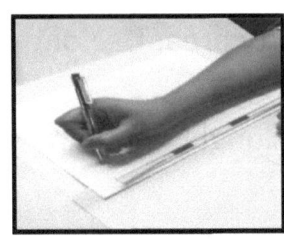

Reference

1. Nicol, M. (2008).*Aseptic Dressing Technique.*www.cetl.org.uk/learning

2. *Ministry Of Health Malaysia, Policies and Procedures on Infection Control", 2nd edition (2010)*

3. *Nursing Division, Ministry Of Health. National Nursing Audit, Version 4(2011)*

CHAPTER 13
Wound Cleansing

Dr Zairudin Abdulah Zawawi

13-1. Definition

Wound cleansing is a process of removing inflammatory contaminants from the wound surface. These contaminants can impede healing and increase risk of infection.

The contaminants are:

1. Necrotic tissues
2. Excess exudates
3. Foreign objects
4. Infected tissues

Solutions used in wound cleansing can be either non-antiseptic or antiseptic.

13-2. Non antiseptic solutions

Non-antiseptic solutions are used to clean wounds. Commonly used non-antiseptic solutions are:

1. **Normal saline**
   - Preferred cleanser for most types of wounds (physiologic and safe)
   - Less effective in dirty and necrotic wounds
   - Not advisable in MRSA and *Pseudomonas* infected wound
   - Once the container is opened, it should be used within 24 hours

2. **Water for irrigation**
   - Less physiologic compared to normal saline but still safe to be used
   - Can be used in MRSA and *Pseudomonas* infected wound

13-3. Antiseptic solutions

Antiseptic solutions are used to clean the wound which are dirty and infected. Commonlly used antiseptic solutions are:

1. ***Chlorhexidine gluconate 1:200 in aqueous solution***
   - Effective against Gram positive bacteria, fungi and also enveloped viruses.
   - Less effective against Gram negative bacteria.
   - Has both bactericidal and bacterostatic action.
   - Readily available in healthcare setting.

2. ***Super-oxidized solution***
   - Good bactericidal, virucidal, fungicidal and spongicidal.
   - Also blocks the inflammatory process.
   - May help in biofilm removal.
   - Two components in this solution are oxidized water and chlorine.
   - The oxidized water is broken down into oxygen, ozone and other oxidized species.
   - Costly.

3. ***Polyhexamethylene biguanide (PHMB) solution***
   - Helps to soften and remove the slough.
   - It can remove and reduce the biofilm formation
   - Less painful.
   - Costly.

These solutions besides painful on application also cause harm to the normal tissues if used as dressing solutions (cytotoxic), however a short term use may be permissible

- Povidone iodine
- Hydrogen peroxide
- Sodium hypochlorite
- Acetic acid
- Eusol

References

1. *Atiyeh BS, Dibo SA, Hayek SN. Wound cleansing, topical antiseptics and wound healing. Int Wound J 2009; 6:420–430*

2. *Ennis WJ, Valdes W, Salzman S, Fishman D, Meneses P. Trauma and wound care. 2004;291-307.*

3. *Chisholm CD, Cordell WH, Rogers K, Woods JR. Comparison of a new pressurized saline canister versus syringe irrigation for laceration cleansing in the emergency department. Ann Emerg Med. Nov 1992;21(11):1364-7. [Medline].*

4. *Watt BE, Proudfoot AT, Vale JA. Hydrogen peroxide poisoning. Toxicol Rev. 2004;23(1):51-7. [Medline].*

5. *Leyden JJ, Bartelt NM. Comparison of topical antibiotic ointments, a wound protectant, and antiseptics for the treatment of human blister wounds contaminated with Staphylococcus aureus. J Fam Pract. Jun 1987;24(6):601-4. [Medline].*

CHAPTER 14: Types of Dressing

Dr Harikrishna K.R Nair

14-1. Dressing Purpose

- Protect wound from trauma and microbial contamination
- Reduce pain
- Maintain temperature & moisture of wound
- Absorb drainage & debride the wound
- Control & Prevent haemorrhage (pressure dressing)
- Provide psychological comfort

Ideal/optimum dressing

- Remove excess exudates
- Waterproof
- Maintain moist wound healing environment
- Trauma protection
- Allows gaseous exchange if appropriate
- Non adherent
- Provide barrier to pathogens
- Safe & easy to use
- Provide thermal insulation

14-2. Dressing Categories

1. Conventional/ Inert
2. Modern/ Advanced/ Active Dressings

Conventional/ Inert

- Gauze –soaked with normal saline / antiseptic
- Gamgee as secondary dressing

Modern/ Advanced/ Active Dressings

DRESSINGS	PURPOSE	ADVANTAGES	DISADVANTAGES	PRACTICAL USAGE
1. **Film**	Protect against contamination and friction Maintain moist surface Prevent evaporation Facilitate assessment	Adherent Transparent with measurement grid Bacterial barrier Waterproof Breathable	Fluid collection Possibility of stripping away newly formed epithelium on removal	Apply the film over the site making sure there is no air under it To remove the film, stretch the film and pull slowly from the edges Frequency of dressing change: 2-5 days depending on the wound
2. **Hydrogel**	Rehydrate, debride and deslough the wound Promote moist healing Cavity filling	Comfortable Provide moist environment and reduce pain Rehydrate eschar Desloughing agent Promotes granulation	Need secondary dressing Maceration of the skin around the wound	Apply the hydrogel on the wound bed as a primary dressing Frequency of dressing change: 2-3 days

DRESSINGS	PURPOSE	ADVANTAGES	DISADVANTAGES	PRACTICAL USAGE
3. Hydro-colloid	Provide moist environment Absorb exudates Bacterial barrier	Cleans and debrides by autolysis Easy to use Cost effective Promotes granulation tissue Effective for low to moderate exuding wounds Waterproof	Unpleasant odour Forms a yellow liquid gel Difficult to use in cavities Maceration of skin around wound	Apply the adhesive side onto the wound without touching the wound bed A yellow liquid is seen after the dressing is left in situ which needs to be cleansed Frequency of dressing change: 2 to 5 days
4. Calcium Alginate	Absorb wound exudates and maintain moisture	Economical and easy to apply Biodegradable Haemostatic properties	Not helpful for dry wounds Need secondary dressing	Available in sheet or rope form Effective to stop bleeding The residue of the biodegradable product has to be washed off during the cleansing process Frequency of dressing change: 2 to 5 days

DRESSINGS	PURPOSE	ADVANTAGES	DISADVANTAGES	PRACTICAL USAGE
5. Foams	Absorbent Cushioning	Conforms to body contours Designed for cavity wounds Highly absorbent Provides protection Bacterial and waterproof	Can adhere to wounds if exudates dries out	Foam dressing is used as a secondary dressing or as cavity fillers. Frequency of dressing change: 2 to 3 days or longer if for offloading
6. Hydrofibre	Manage heavy exuding wounds Maintains moist healing environment	Longer wear time Comfortable and non traumatic upon removal Reduce risk of maceration Can be use on infected wounds	Not helpful for dry wounds Needs secondary dressings	The hydrofibre will become gel-like layer which can be easily removed Frequency of dressing change: 2 to 5 days
7. Charcoal	Odour absorbent	Reduces odour	Needs secondary dressing	Frequency of dressing change: 2 days
8. Silver	To reduce bacterial bioburden in infected wounds	Locally acting No known resistance Bactericidal	Some silver dressings do discolour the wound	Place the dressing with the side with silver facing the wound bed Frequency of dressing change: 2 to 3 days

DRESSINGS	PURPOSE	ADVANTAGES	DISADVANTAGES	PRACTICAL USAGE
9. Multi-function dressing (Polymeric membrane dressing)	To manage moisture imbalance (from dry to moderate)	Antiseptic property Has surfactant which helps to cleanse the wound when it is applied Offloading property	Not for heavily exudative wounds.	Frequency of dressing change: 2 to 5 days
10. Composite dressing (combination of 2 or more dressing materials)	According to components of the materials	multifunction	Same as individual components listed above	Frequency of dressing change: 2 to 5 days
11. Other advanced dressings	Not widely used – some may be used in specialised center e.g Collagen, matrix and regenerative dressings, cultured epidermis, growth factors, stem cells			

Points to remember:
- Know your dressing material well and use it judiciously
- All wounds need to be cleansed thoroughly before applying any types of dressing materials

References

1. Harikrishna K.R.Nair. Compendium of Wound Care Dressings in Malaysia. Volume 1 (2012)

2. Harikrishna K.R.Nair. Compendium of Wound Care Dressings in Malaysia. Volume 2 (2013)

CHAPTER 15

Wound Debridement

Dr.Mohamed Yusof Hj Abdul Wahab / Dr.Harikrishna K.R Nair/ Dr.Zairudin Abdullah Zawawi

15-1. Introduction

It is a process of removal of non viable tissue and contaminants from a wound to promote healing.

Methods of debridement:

- Surgical
- Autolytic
- Enzymatic
- Mechanical
- Biological
- Hydrostatic

15-2. Surgical Debridement

Removal of necrotic tissue by sharp debridement using a scalpel, scissors, curette, Humby knife, electrical dermatome or other instrument to cut necrotic tissue from a wound as to prepare the wound bed for optimum healing.

Indications

1. Extensive Devitalized Tissue
2. Signs of advancing soft tissue infections or sepsis
3. Presence of thick adherent eschar
4. Callous formation

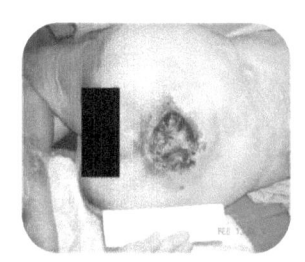

Figure 15.1 Thick Eschar

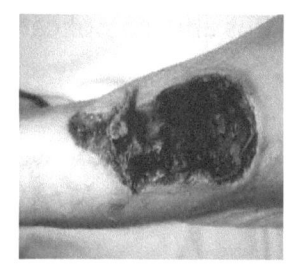

Figure 15.2 Extensive devitalized tissue

SECTION C: PRACTICAL ASPECT IN WOUNDCARE | 137

> **Specialist consultation may be required in the following condition:**
> 1. Vascular insufficiency (lack of blood flow impairs healing)
> 2. Gangrenous wound
> 3. Unidentifiable structures (risk of injuring vital structures eg. nerves)
> 4. Coagulopathy (risk of bleeding. Debridement better handled in tertiary centres)
> 5. Stable heel ulcer (if firmly adherent, lack of inflammation, lack of drainage, eschar that does not feel soft and boggy)
> 6. Fungating/ malignant wounds (treatment may involve extensive dissection or removal of entire anatomical part. Debridement is non-curative)
> 7. Necrotic tissues near and/or involving neurovascular structures
> 8. Wounds of hand and face

Assessment of Wounds Indicated for Surgical Debridement

All wounds intended for debridement must be assessed with regards to its suitability for surgical debridement. The following factors may be used as a guideline:-

1. The nature of the necrotic or ischemic tissue and the best debridement procedure to follow
2. The risk of spreading infection and the use of antibiotics
3. The presence of underlying medical conditions causing the wound
4. The extent of ischemia in the wound tissues
5. The location of the wound in the body
6. The type of analgesia to be used during the procedure
7. Possible complications

Basic Principles of Surgical Debridement

1. Debride in stages to minimize damage to healthy tissue.

2. Staying within a given facial plane during debridement avoids spreading bacteria into the lower layers. If a fascial plane is reached, one must stop and reassess the situation to determine if whether deeper debridement is needed.

3. Small bleeders can be stopped with the application of pressure while large bleeders require diathermy or ligation of vessels.

4. Pain control during debridement may be achieved using oral analgesics, topical analgesics, intravenous or intramuscular drugs and regional or general anesthesia (refer chapter on pain management)

Viable vs Non-viable Tissue

The following table describes the intra-operative observation according to tissue differentiation.

Tissue	Non viable	Viable
Fat	Dull, Gray/brown to black	Shiny yellow
Fascia	Dull, Gray/brown to black	Glistening White

Tissue	Non viable	Viable
Muscle	Dark red/brown to gray	Dull red Possible contraction if pinched
All tissue	No sensation Avascular- no bleeding Frequently foul odor	Good vascularity – punctate bleeding Little or no odor

* *Periosteum deserves special mention. Cardinal rule is to leave periosteum alone as it will granulate. It also will accept skin grafts in contrast to cortical bone which will not.*

Instruments for Surgical Debridement

- Instruments used for the procedure may include scissors, forceps, scalpel, curette, Humby knife, electrical dermatome and hemostats.
- Scalpels should be used sparingly, they can cause too much inadvertent cutting
- Curved scissors are preferred to flat scissors for two reasons – when cutting with the tips there is less risk of accidental injury by the tip occurs and when cutting with the tips down, cutting can be performed in a tighter area. Easily controlled instrument.
- A curette can scoop underneath adherent necrotic tissue, avoiding the difficult manipulation of scissors and forceps. However, it is difficult to control the depth of debridement while using this instrument.

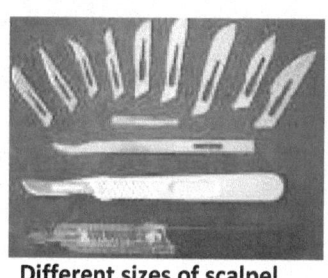

Different sizes of scalpel

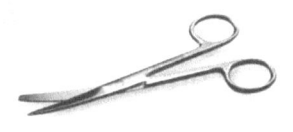

Curved scissor

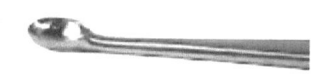

Curette

15-3. Autolytic Debridement

Definition

- The process by which the wound bed utilizes phagocytes and proteolytic enzymes to remove non-viable tissue
- This process can be promoted and enhanced by maintaining a moist wound environment.

Mode of Action

Hydrogel

- Gently rehydrates dry necrotic tissue
- Provides moist wound healing environment
- Softens necrotic tissue

15-4. Enzymatic Debridement

- The use of topically applied enzymatic agents is to stimulate the breakdown of non-viable tissue
- Faster debridement process compared to autolytic
- Examples are Clostridiopeptidase A, honey and fibrinolysin with DNAse

15-5. Mechanical Debridement

1. Wet To Dry Gauze
   Usage of gauze to peel the necrotic tissue from the wound bed
   This procedure can be very painful

2. Scrubbing
   Using the blunt edge of the scalpel or forceps to remove biofilm and debris

3. Whirlpool
   This utilizes low pressure water force to cleanse and debride the wound bed. Less harmful to normal cells.

4. Wound Irrigation
   Using non antiseptic cleansing solution to irrigate and debride the wound.

15-6. Biological Debridement

Maggot Debridement Therapy (MDT) is one of the modality in managing wounds. There are two species which are used in MDT i.e Lucilia cuprina (Malaysia and tropical country) and Lucilia sericata (temperate country).

Definition of MDT:
- The use of STERILE maggots for the debridement of wounds in humans
- This therapy is :
    1. Hypoallergenic
    2. Non-invasive
    3. Effective

Mechanisms of action:
- Remove slough
    - proteases dissolve necrotic and infective material (Vistnes 1981, Constable 1994, Case 1994)
- Stimulate wound healing
    - promote granulation & epithelialization (Horobin 2003, 2006, Nigam 2006)
- Disinfect the wound
    - ingest bacteria e.g Proteus sp. (Klaus L 2003)
    - pH changes
    - antibacterial substance (<1kD) (Kerridge A 2005)

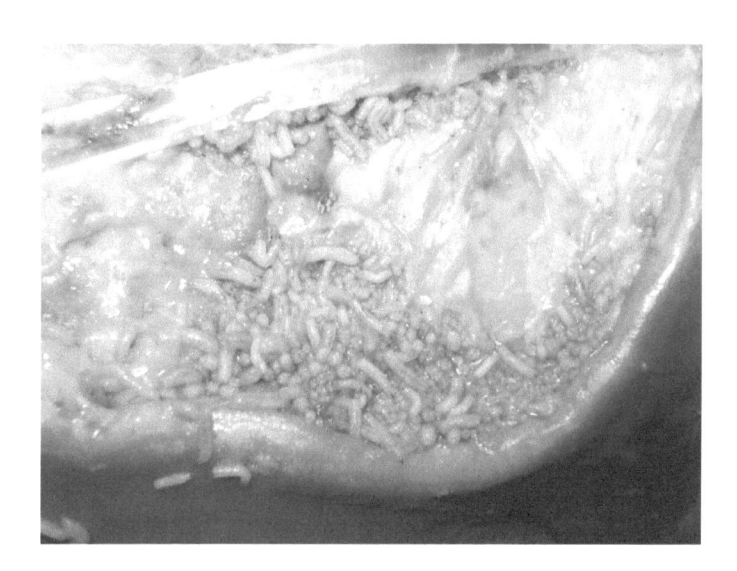

Contraindications:

1. Wounds needing urgent debridement
2. Bleeding wounds
3. Poor vascularity
4. Abscesses
5. Entomophobia (*an abnormal and persistent fear of insects*)
6. Fistula, joints, deep cavities
7. Near neurovascular bundles

Hydrostatic Debridement

HIGH POWER HYDROSTATIC DEBRIDER

- Powered instrument for surgical debridement of wounds
- Excise tissue with a stream of saline
- Combined localised vacuum removing excised tissue immediately
- Holds, cuts and removes tissue at the same time
- Hydrostatic debridement is more precise and more selective than a scalpel
- Enable surgeon to precisely target (through different power settings) and removes devitalised tissue and contaminants and at the same time preserves collateral healthy tissue

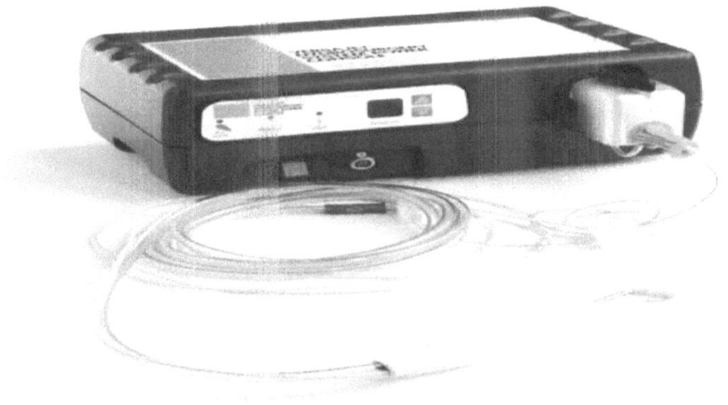

Figure 15.4 High Power Hydrostatic Debrider

> **Points to remember:**
> - Wound debridement is paramount to create a stable wound

References

1. *Comprehensive Wound Management 2nd ed; Glenn L.Irion , Phd. PT.CWS*
2. *Sharp Debridement; Vince Lepak, PT, MPH, CWS*
3. *Loehne, H.B. (2002). Wound debridement and irrigation. In L.C.Kloth and J.M. McCulloch*
4. *Bergstrom,N.,Bennet,M.A.,Carlson,C.E.,et al(1994).Treatment of pressure ulcers.*
5. *Leaper D (2002) Sharp technique for wound debridement World Wide Wounds December*
6. *NICE (2001) Guidelines on Pressure ulcer risk assessment and prevention NICE London*
7. *Guidelines for the Assessment and Management of Wounds(2006);NHS*

CHAPTER 16 Adjunctive Teatment
a) Honey Dressing

Dr. Mohamad Izani Ibrahim

16a-1. Introduction

1. Honey has been rediscovered to have medicinal value in treating wounds. Numerous studies have compared honey with other modern dressings in managing various type of wounds.

2. Honey is mainly used to promote granulation and epithelization of a wound for secondary intention healing or to be followed by further surgical procedure for soft tissue coverage, e.g: split skin graft, full thickness skin graft, flaps.

3. Honey has antibacterial effects which are attributed to its high osmolarity, low pH, hydrogen peroxide content, and presence of other uncharacterized compounds.

4. There are various types of honey in the market. They consist of raw honey, commercial honey and therapeutic honey.

    - Raw honey
        - enzymes is maintained
        - Risk of having clostridial spores.

    - Commercial honey
        - Enzymes are destroyed by pasteurization
        - Still have the properties of osmotic effects

    - Therapeutic honey
        - Is the most suitable to be used in wound dressing.
        - Prepared specifically for medical use and are sterilized through an irradiation process that does not damage their constituents
        - However it is more expensive
        - Also available in the form of pre-impregnated dressing pads

Possible general benefits and functions of honey are:

- antimicrobial property
- promote enzymatic debridement
- deodorize malodorous wounds
- stimulate growth of wound tissues to accelerate healing
- stimulate anti-inflammatory activity that reduces pain, edema and exudates
- minimizes hypertrophic scar
- promote moist wound healing
- contains low level hydrogen peroxide which stimulates fibroblast proliferation and angiogenesis

Adverse effects (rare)

It consists of:

a) Allergy

b) Transient stinging sensation in some patients – mainly in wounds with severe inflammatory process.

Contraindication for honey dressing

a) History of allergy and sensitive to bee sting, honey products.

b) Dry, necrotic wounds- honey can cause further drying of the wound.

16a-2. Principles of Honey dressing

a) Application of honey- it is best to spread the honey on a dressing and apply the honey directly onto the wound.

b) Dressing pads preimpregnated with honey are commercially available and provide an effective and less messy alternative.

c) The amount of honey to be used depends on the amount of fluid exudates of the wound as well as the wound size.

d) Large amount of exudates needs more honey to be applied. Typically 20ml of honey is used on a 10cm x 10cm dressing.

e) Frequency of dressing: once daily up to every 3 days. The frequency of dressing changes depends on how rapidly the honey is being diluted by the exudates. The more the exudates the more the frequency.

f) In high exudates wounds, the frequency of dressing will be less frequent as the honey starts to work on healing the wound.

g) On changing of the honey dressing, the removal of the dressing should be easy. If not, this shows that the amount of honey or frequency of dressing is inadequate and should be increased.

h) Occlusive (waterproof) or absorbent secondary dressings help to prevent honey oozing out from the wound (occlusive dressing better as it keeps more of the honey in contact with the wound)

i) Pressure bandaging is used over honey dressing for varicose ulcers.

Steps in Performing Honey Dressing

1.	Prepare equipments a) honey b) gauze/cotton c) occlusive dressing(if use) d) dressing set	
2.	Wound cleansing should follow standard procedure mentioned in wound cleansing section Application of honey- it is best to spread the honey on a dressing and apply the honey directly onto the wound Dressing pads preimpregnated with honey are commercially available and provide an effective and less messy alternative	

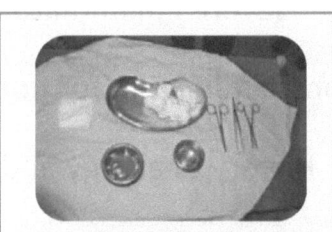

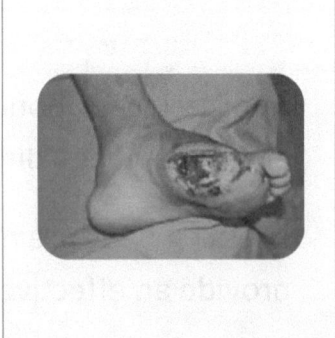

3.	Estimate amount of honey according to wound size and exudates. The amount of honey depends on the amount of fluid exudates of the wound as well as the wound size. Large amount of exudates needs more honey to be applied. Typically 20ml of honey is used on a 10cm x 10cm dressing. Dressing frequency can be as frequent as once daily up to every 3 days. It depends on how rapidly the honey is being diluted by the exudates. The more the exudates the more the frequency.	
4.	Soak gauze/cotton into the honey using dressing forceps	
5.	Apply the gauze/cotton soaked honey onto the wound up to the edges. It can also be applied onto the surrounding skin to reduce local inflammation. On changing of the honey dressing, the removal of the dressing should be easy. If not, this shows that the amount of honey or frequency of dressing is inadequate and should be increased	
6.	Apply several more layers of gauze onto this gauze soaked hone. Apply bandage on the dressing or an occlusive dressing. Occlusive (waterproof) or absorbent secondary dressings help to prevent honey oozing out from the wound (occlusive dressing better as it keeps more of the honey in contact with the wound). Pressure bandaging is used over honey dressing for varicose ulcers.	

> **Point to Remember:**
>
> - Although it has debridement activity, its main functions are to promote granulation and epithelization of a wound.
>
> - Any type of honey can be used, but the most suitable is the therapeutic honey.
>
> - Honey dressing is not a substitute for a proper surgical debridement.

References

1. Blomfield R. Honey for decubitus ulcers. J Am Med Assoc ;224(6):905, 1973.

2. Bulman MW. Honey as a surgical dressing. Middlesex Hosp J ;55:188-189, 1955.

3. Chung Ly, Schmidt Rj, Hamlyn Pf, Sagar Bf, Andrews Am, Turner Td. Biocompatibility of potential wound management products: hydrogen peroxide generation by fungal chitin/chitosans and their effects on the proliferation of murine L929 fibroblasts in culture. Journal of Biomedical Material Research 39, 300-307, 1998.

4. DUNFORD CE, HANANO R. Acceptability to patients of a honey dressing for non-healing venous leg ulcers. Journal of Wound Care, 13, 193-7, 2004.

5. Efem SEE. Clinical observations on the wound healing properties of honey. Br J Surg; 75:679-681, 1988.

6. Hutton DJ. Treatment of pressure sores. Nurs Times ;62(46):1533-1534, 1966.

7. Lay-flurrie K. Honey in wound care: effects, clinical application and patient benefits. Br J Nursing 17(11): S30–6, 2008.

8. Molan PC. The antibacterial activity of honey.Bee World ;73(1):5-28, 1992.

9. Molan PC. The antibacterial properties of honey. 5. Chem NZ ;59:10-14, 1995.

10. MOLAN, PC Potential of honey in the treatment of wounds and burns. American Journal of Clinical Dermatology, 2, 13-9, 2001.

11. Molan PC. Mode of action. In: White RJ, Cooper RA, Molan PC (eds) Honey: A Modern Wound Management Product. Wounds UK, Aberdeen, 2005.

12. MOLAN, PC. The evidence supporting the use of honey as a wound dressing. International Journal of Lower Extremity Wounds 5, 40-54, 2006.

13. Ndayisaba G, Bazira L, Habonimana E, Muteganya D. Clinical and bacteriological results in wounds treated with honey. J Orthop Surg;7(2):202-204, 1993.

14. Sadagatullah Abdul Nawfar, Chung Seng Han, Mohammad Paiman and Mohd Iskandar. A Randomized Control Trial Comparing the Effects of Manuka Honey and Tualang Honey on Wound Granulation of Post Debridement Diabetic Foot Wounds Journal of ApiProduct and ApiMedical Science 3 (1): 18 - 25 ,2011.

15. Subrahmanyam M. Topical application of honey in treatment of burns. Br J Surj;78(4);497-498, 1991.

16. Wood B, Rademaker M, Molan PC. Manuka honey, a low cost leg ulcer dressing. N Z Med J; 110:107, 1997.

CHAPTER 16

Adjunctive Treatment
b) Hyperbaric Oxygen Therapy (HBOT) in Wound Care

Dr. Mohd. Zamzuri bin Mohd. Zain/ Col. (Dr.) Muhd. Yusof bin Abu Bakar

16b-1. Introduction

- Intermittently breathing pure (100%) oxygen at greater than ambient pressure
- Oxygen as a drug and hyperbaric chamber as a dosing device
- Elevating tissue oxygen tension is the primary effect

HBOT may be used as an Adjunct Therapy in the Following Condition

- Diabetic Foot Ulcer
- Osteoradionecrosis of Mandible
- Clostridial myositis and myonecrosis (gas gangrene)
- Crush injury, compartment syndrome, acute traumatic ischaemias
- Enhance healing of wounds (acute and chronic)
- Necrotizing fasciitis
- Chronic osteomyelitis
- Thermal burns

*Currently Health Technology Assessment (HTA) Ministry of Health Malaysia recommends the usage of HBOT in Diabetic Foot Ulcer and Osteoradionecrosis of Mandible

16b-2. Mechanism of Action

- Angiogenesis in ischaemic tissues
- Both bacteriostatic and bactericidal actions
- Inhibition of *Clostridium perfringens* alpha toxin synthesis
- Vasoconstriction
- Enhancing Collagen synthesis
- Leukocyte oxidative killing

Treatment Process

- Place patient in chamber
- Type A, Multiplace (2-14 patients) or Type B, Monoplace (1 person) chamber

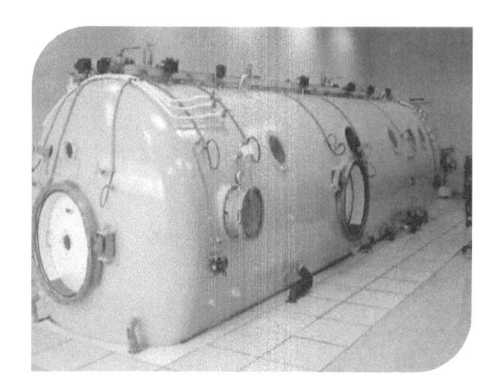

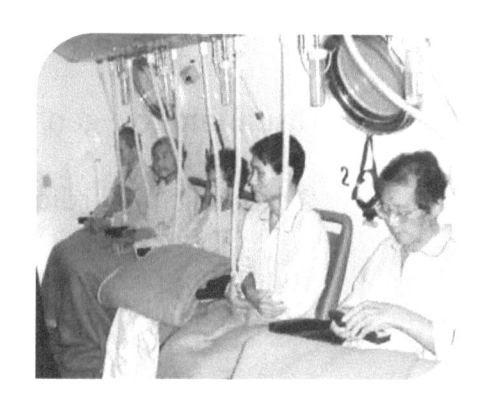

Figure 16b.1 Type A - Multiplace chamber

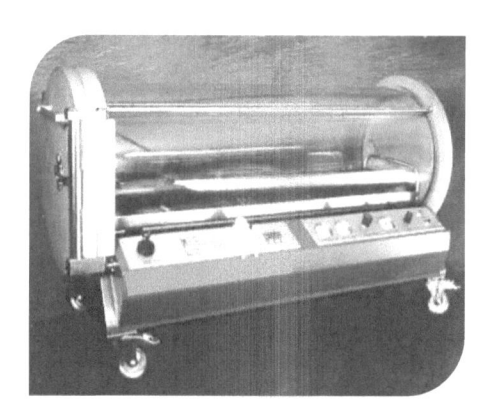

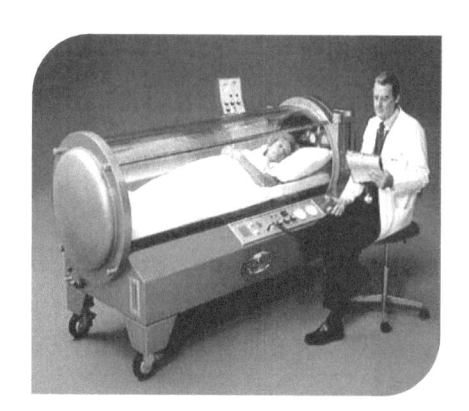

Figure 16b.2 Type B - Monoplace chamber

- Pressures applied inside the chamber are usually 2-3 times ambient atmosphere pressure.
- Treatments may take 2-8 hours
- Beware of any possible complications

16b-3. Absolute Contraindication

- Untreated pneumothorax (barotrauma)
- Patient on drugs/medication as follows
    - Bleomycin (intestitial pneumonitis)
    - Cisplatin (impaired wound healing)
    - Disulfiram (oxygen toxicity)
    - Doxorubicin (cardiotoxicity)
    - Sulfamylon (impaired wound healing)

16b-4. Relative Contraindication

- Asthma (may cause pneumothorax)
- Claustrophobia (may cause anxiety)
- Congenital spherocytosis (may cause severe hemolysis)
- COPD (may cause loss of hypoxic drive leads to dyspnea)
- Eustachian tube blockage (may cause tympanic membrane rupture)
- High fever (may cause seizure)
- Pacemaker (may cause malfunction)
- Epidural pain pump (may cause deformation)
- Pregnancy (unknown effect)
- Seizures (may cause lower threshold)
- URTI (may cause barotrauma)

16b-5. Example of chronic non healing diabetic foot ulcers treated with HBOT

Courtesy from Col (Dr) Muhd. Yusof

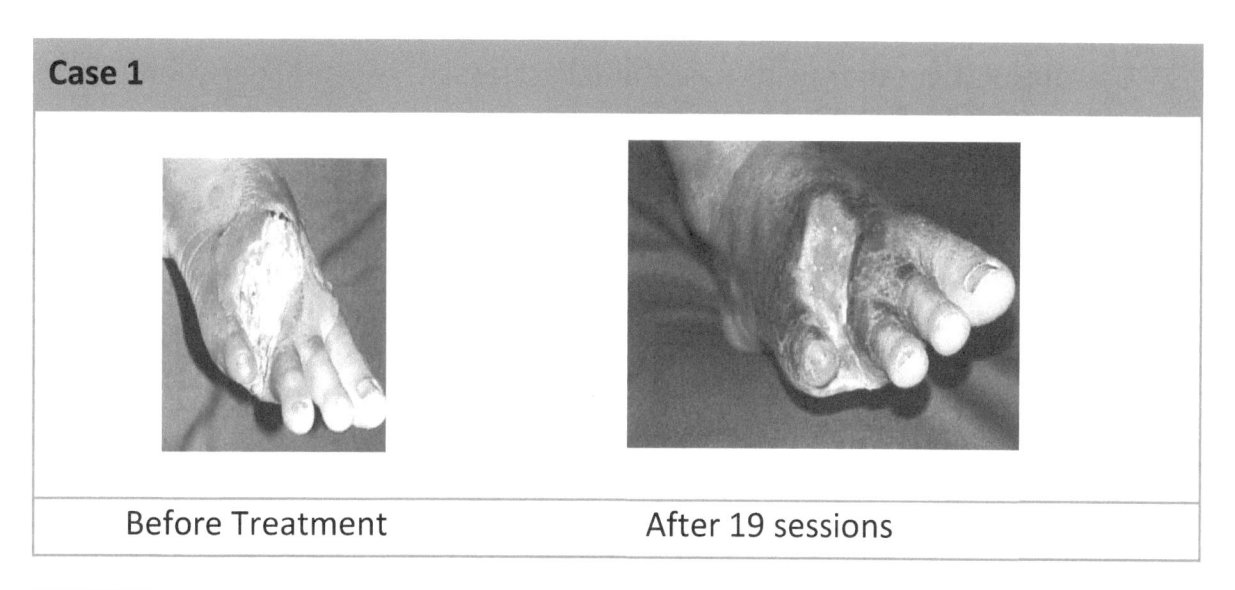

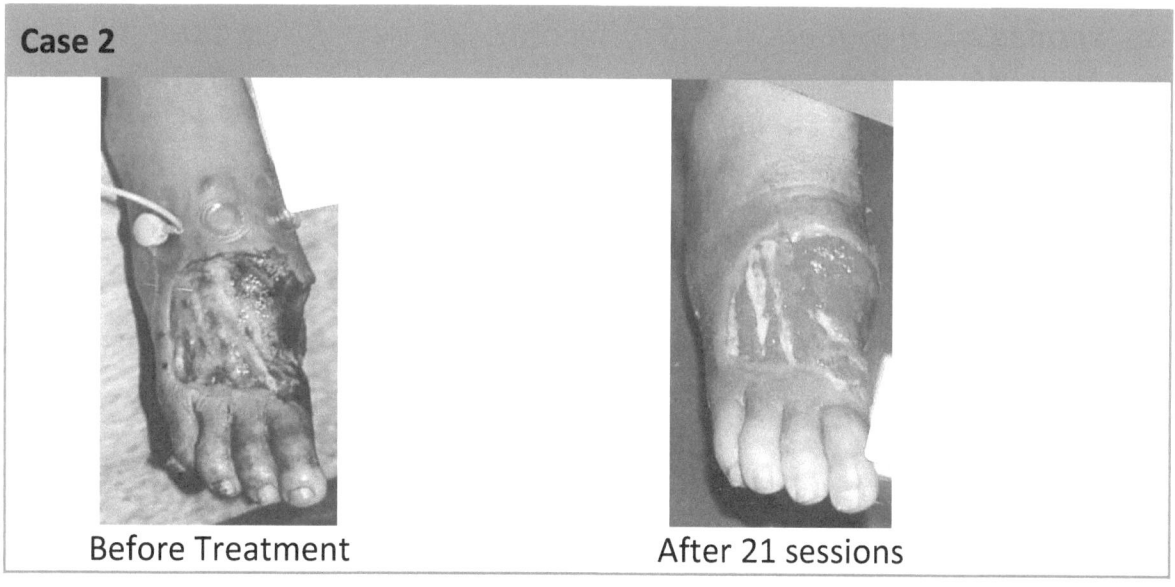

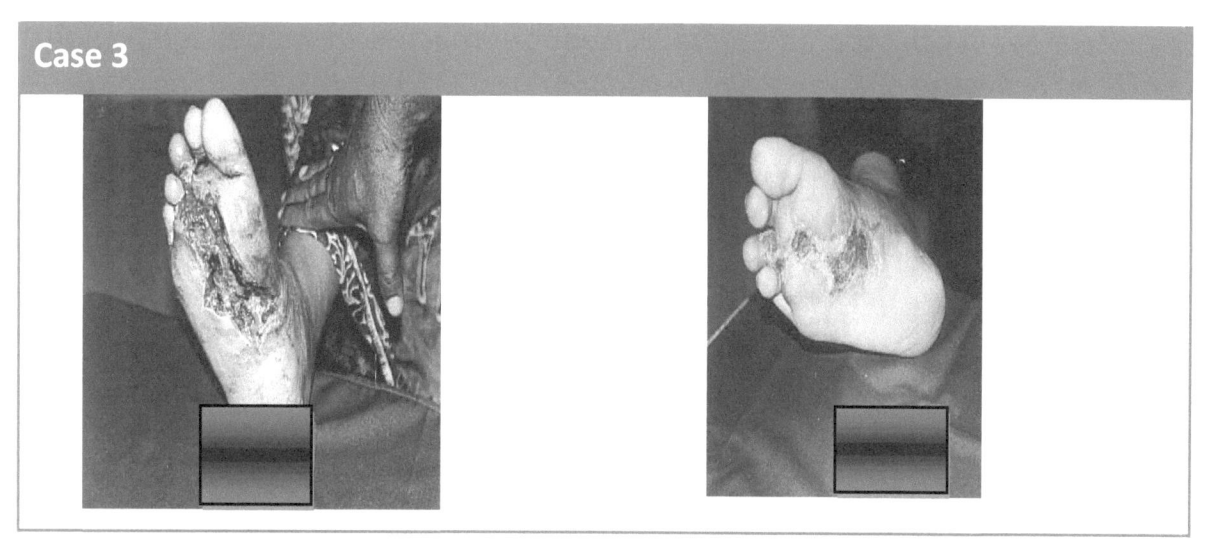

Case 1

| Before Treatment | After 19 sessions |

Case 2

| Before Treatment | After 21 sessions |

Case 3

16b-6. Emerging Concepts of HBOT

- Increasing interest and research regarding HBOT as adjunct treatment in wound healing

- Use of HBOT in other fields e.g. multiple sclerosis, cerebral palsy, and vegetative coma is also being explored

> **Points to remember:**
> - HBOT is used only as **adjunctive treatment**.

References

1. Anne M Eskes, Dirk T Ubbink, Maarten J Lubbers, Cees Lucas, Hester Vermeulen. Hyperbaric Oxygen Therapy: Solution for Difficult to Heal Acute Wounds? Systematic Review. World Journal of Surgery. New York: Mar 2011. Vol. 35, Iss. 3; pg. 535

2. Anonymous How to manage the diabetic foot.. Nursing Times. London: Apr 02, 2011.

3. Overview of Hyperbaric Oxygen Therapy (Medscape)

4. Rena G Diem. Pearls for Practice: Hyperbaric Oxygen Therapy (HBOT) and Heel Ulcers. Ostomy Wound Management. King of Prussia: Sep 2011. Vol.57, Iss. 9;pg. 8

5. Renée A Beach, Adam J Mamelak 'New' approaches to venous congestion.. Expert Review of Dermatology. London: Dec 2010. Vol. 5, Iss. 6; pg. 589

6. James Wright. Hyperbaric Oxygen Therapy for wound healing., e-medicine. New York. May 2011

CHAPTER 16

Management of Acute Wound
c) Negative Pressure Wound Therapy (NPWT)

Dr. Normala Hj. Basiron

16c-1. Introduction

NPWT provides a new paradigm that can be used in concert with a wide variety of standard existing techniques in wound management. The ease of technique and a high rate of success have encouraged its adaptation by various disciplines.

16c-2. What is NPWT?

NPWT is a recent technique which facilitates wound treatment utilizing subatmospheric pressure. It consists of placing an open cell wound interface e.g. sponge/gauze directly on the wound surface and covering it with an occlusive film. Negative pressure (below that of ambient pressure) is applied to the entire wound surface so that the wound interface contents move toward the pump.

Contents of NPWT dressing pack

a. Sterile open cell wound interface of small, medium and large sizes.
b. Pliable vacuum tubing.
c. An occlusive adhesive transparent dressing.
d. Canister (collection chamber with connecting tubing).
e. Vacuum pump.

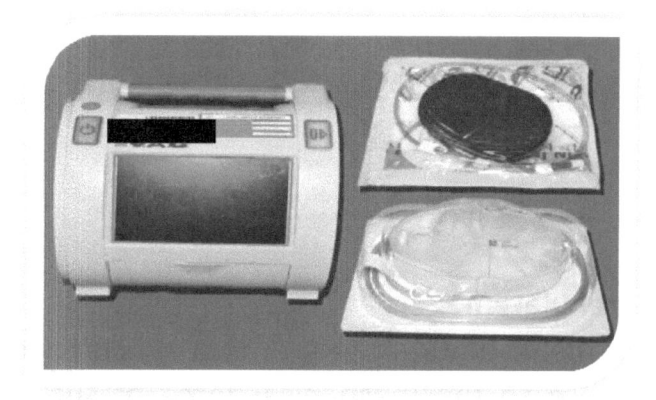

Figure 16c.1 NPWT dressing pack

16C-3. How NPWT works?

1. **Provides a closed and moist wound healing environment.**
   - Helps encourage granulation tissue growth at wound site, and helps reduce contamination from outside bacteria
   - Reduces cell death caused by dehydration

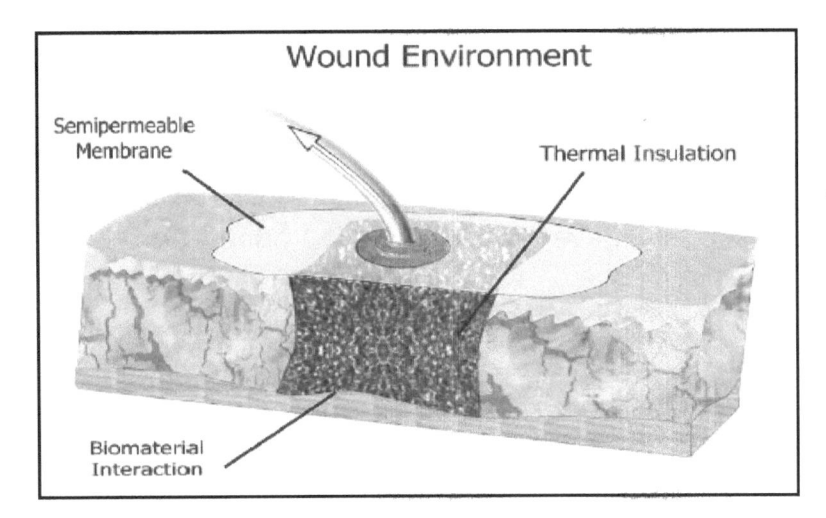

Figure 16c.2 Wound environment

The NPWT device keeps the wound moist and warm compared to dry dressings that allow the wound to dry out and form a scab. The device also acts as an insulating layer.

2. **Decreases wound volume.**
   - Draws the wound together, approximating the wound edges.

3. **Removes excess fluids that can inhibit wound healing.**
   - Helps decrease bacterial colonization at wound site.

4. **Helps remove interstitial fluid.**
   - Can positively influence reduction in oedema, helping improve blood flow to the wound.

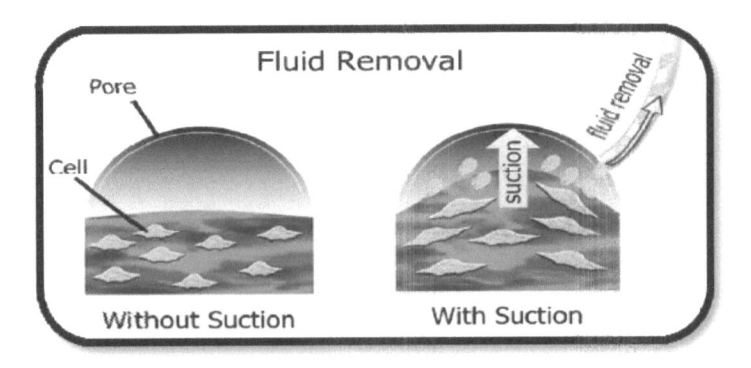

Figure 16c.3 Fluid removal

The foam distributes the vacuum evenly throughout the wound and allow for transport of extracellular fluid to wound surface.

5. **Promotes granulation.**
   - Movement and growth of tissue surrounding the wound in response to the mechanical force of suction pressure (increase mitosis)

SECTION C: PRACTICAL ASPECT IN WOUNDCARE | 158

16c-4. Indications of NPWT

1. Huge, clean and/ or exudative wound while waiting for definitive wound closure.
2. Fixation of skin grafts (mesh-grafts) and tissue flaps

16c-5. Contraindications of NPWT

1. Clotting disorders (risk of bleeding).
2. Necrotic wound bed or eschar (barrier to new tissue growth).
3. Untreated infection (due to deep extension of a potential infectious focus, simple surface treatment is unlikely to be successful).
4. Neoplastic tissue in the wound area (may promote neoplastic tissue growth).

16c-6. How to Apply NPWT?

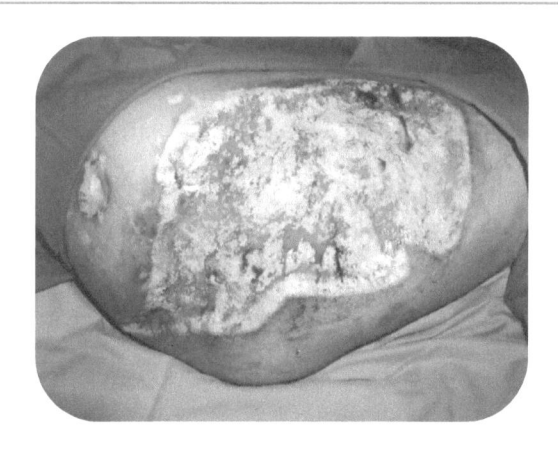

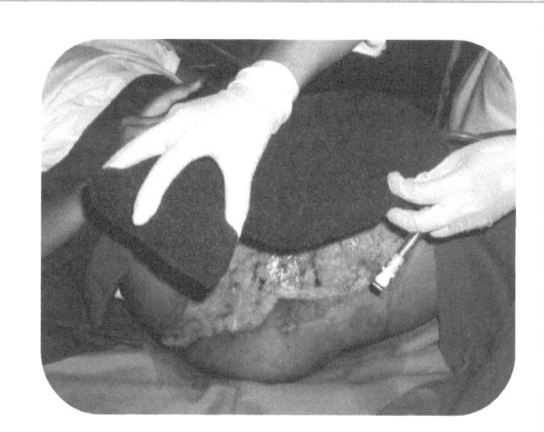

- Cut wound interface to fit the shape of wound
- Place wound interface on wound bed till flushed with edges
- Place vented end of pliable vacuum tubing flush with wound interface

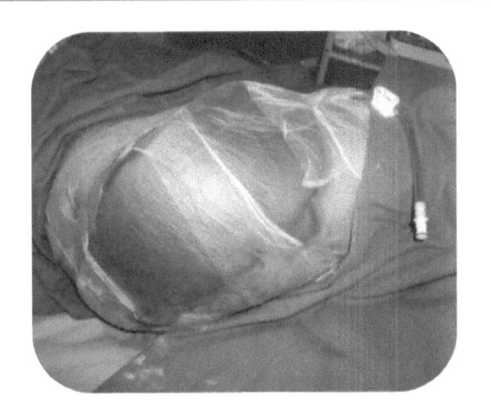

- Cover wound interface and tubing with occlusive adhesive dressing
- Ensure tight seal

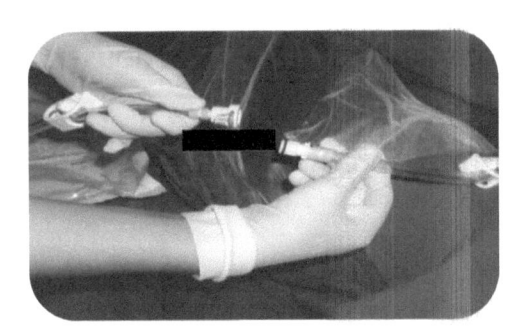

- Connect open end of tubing to canister on vacuum pump

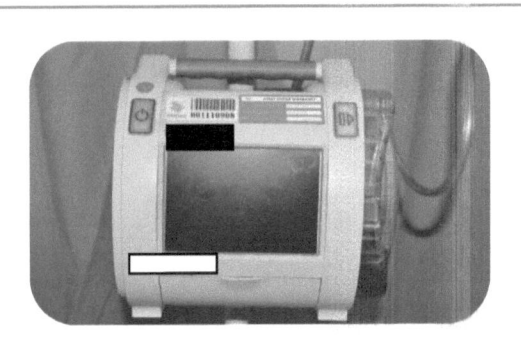

- Program prescribed amount of pressure and suction interval

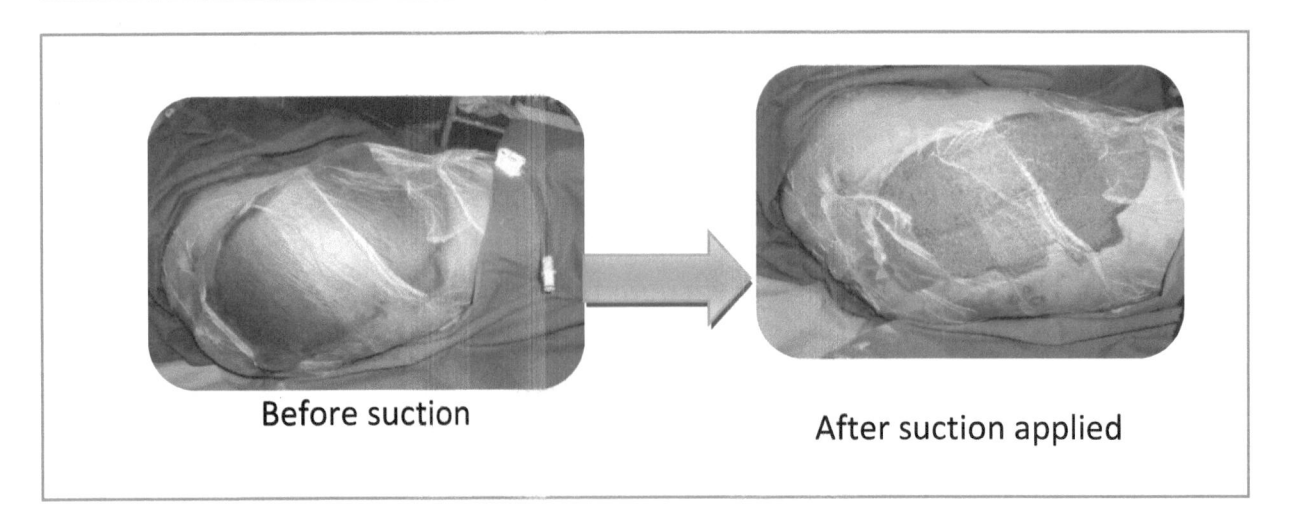

Before suction → After suction applied

SECTION C: PRACTICAL ASPECT IN WOUNDCARE | 160

Recommended NPWT settings:	
Mesh grafts	50 – 75 mmHg of continuous negative pressure for 4 – 5 days
Pressure ulcers and acute wounds	125 mmHg continuous negative pressure for 48 hours, later switched to intermittent intervals (5 minutes on and 2 minutes off)
Chronic ulcers (venous stasis, arterial insufficiency and neuropathies)	Continuous therapy at 50 – 75 mmHg
Compromised tissue flaps	125 mmHg of continuous therapy till base adhesion achieved
NPWT dressing change	3 – 5 days interval or depending on the amount or characteristic of fluid withdrawn as well as the surrounding skin appearance e.g. inflamed, macerated, etc

The technical advances in the new generation NPWT devices will have different modification and specification in their applications to overcome the possible side effects. e.g. light weight computerized battery devices, the type of wound interface, non adherent dressing over the wound before applying wound interface and negative pressure, setting options for automatic instillation system, etc.

16c-7. Complications of NPWT

Complication is infrequent if patients are properly selected and treated. Few reported complications include:

- Toxic shock syndrome.
- Wound infection caused by anaerobes.
- Loss of blood and fluid.

16c-8. Side Effects of NPWT

1. Ingrowth of granulation tissue into the foam.
2. Pain associated with the effects of suction and dressing changes.
3. Maceration and pressure damage to skin areas adjacent to the wound.
4. Reduction in perfusion caused by pressure on small caliber vessels.

> **Points to remember:**
> - NPWT is only an adjunct to the management of chronic, acute and difficult wounds and it is not a panacea.
> - NPWT prepares wound bed for a greater chance of successful closure.
> - NPWT does not replace surgical procedures

References

1. *Attinger, C. E., Janis, J. E., Steinberg, J., et al. Clinical approach to wounds: Debridement and wound bed preparation including the use of dressings and wound-healing adjuvants. PRS. June supplement 2006. 117: 72s-109s, 2006*

2. *Argenta, L. C., Morykwas, M. K., Marks, M. W., et al. Vacuum-Assisted Closure: State of clinic art. PRS. June supplement 2006. 117: 127s-142s, 2006*

3. *Willy, C. The theory and practice of Vacuum therapy. Scientific basis, indications for use, case reports, practical advice. Lindqvist book-publishing ulm 2006, Germany.*

4. *Peinemann F, Sauerland S: Negative pressure wound therapy – systemic review of randomized controlled trials. Dtsch Arztebl Int 2011; 108(22): 381-9.*

CHAPTER 17
Algorithm for Wound Care Treatment

Dr Mohammad Anwar Hau Abdullah

The algorithm is theoretically developed based on T.I.M.E. concept; it intends to be a simple quick practical guide in general principles of wound bed preparation and wound care; for those health care providers who are not familiar with wound management.

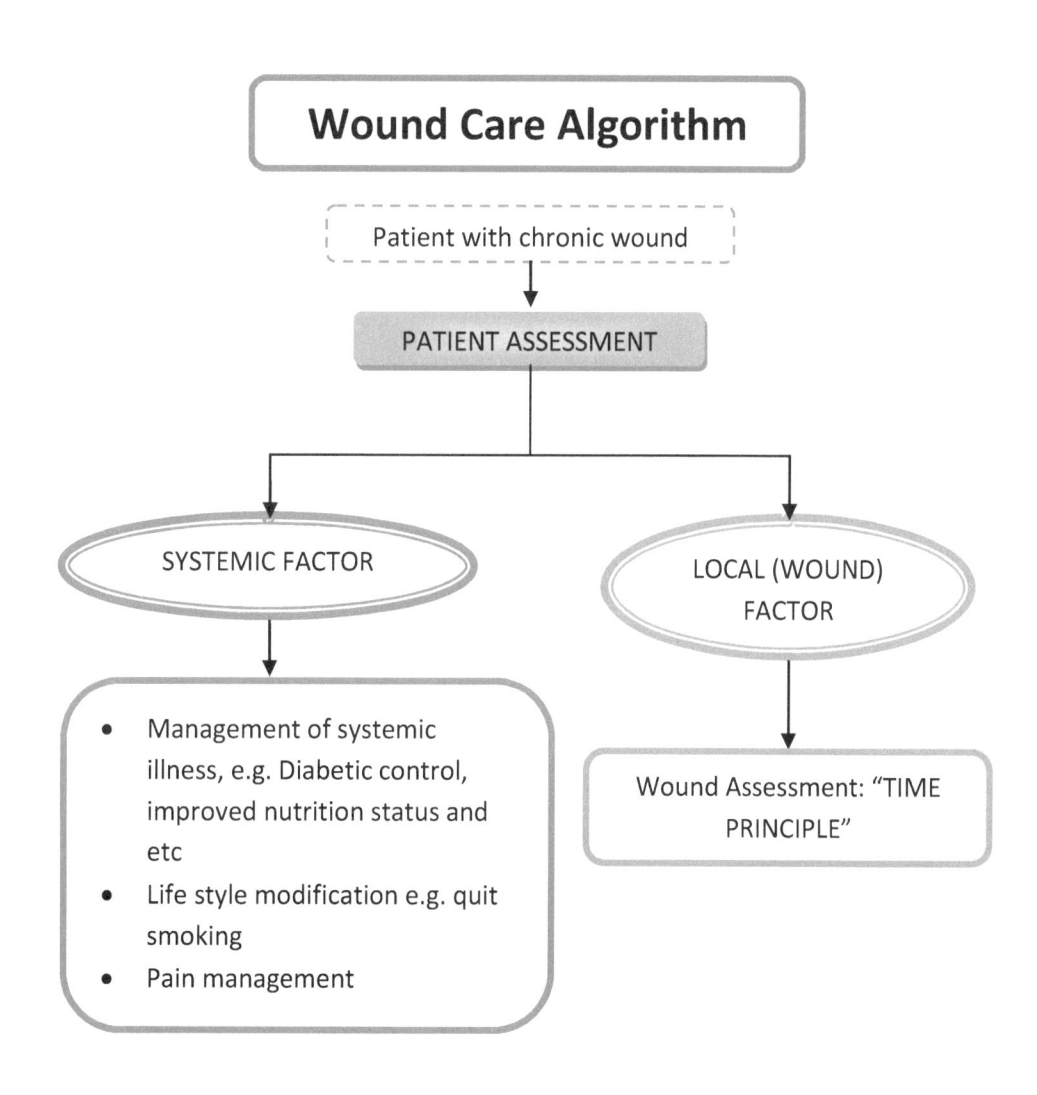

Wound Care Algorithm

Patient with chronic wound
↓
PATIENT ASSESSMENT
├── SYSTEMIC FACTOR
│   - Management of systemic illness, e.g. Diabetic control, improved nutrition status and etc
│   - Life style modification e.g. quit smoking
│   - Pain management
└── LOCAL (WOUND) FACTOR
    - Wound Assessment: "TIME PRINCIPLE"

SECTION C: PRACTICAL ASPECT IN WOUNDCARE | 163

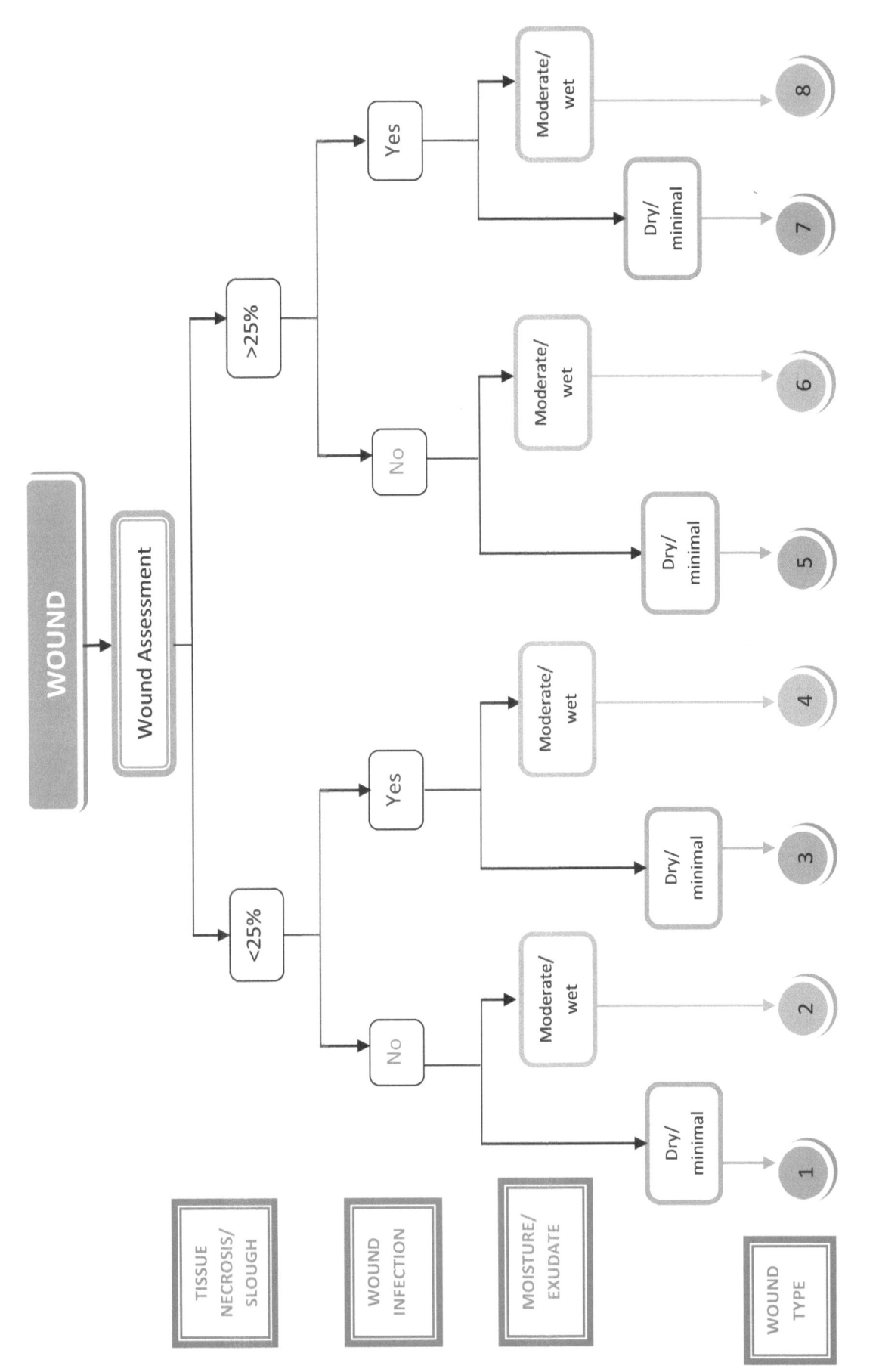

Figure 17.1 Wound Care Algorithm

SECTION C: PRACTICAL ASPECT IN WOUNDCARE | 164

Treatment recommendation based on the flow chart of Wound Care Algorithm:

WOUND TYPE	Wound description	Dressing material suggested/recommended *(refer to chapter on dressing materials)*	Antibiotic	Surgical procedure suggested/recommended
1	Clean, healthy granulating wound	All types of dressing material except, silver, charcoal and special advanced dressing materials.	No	1. Ready for secondary wound closure 2. If the wound is small, continue dressing till the wound heals by secondary intention 3. Frequency of wound dressing varies depending on type of wound and also dressing material used
2	Clean and wet wound	1. Foam 2. Alginate 3. Hydrofiber 4. Polymeric membrane	May or may not, based on the underlying cause.	1. Find underlying cause 2. Treat underlying cause if necessary
3	Dry, infected wound with < 25% slough/necrotic tissue (most likely vascular in origin)	1. Tulle 2. Hydrogel 3. Hydrocolloid 4. Silver dressing 5. Iodine base dressing	Yes, based on C&S report of infected tissue	1. Debridement may be needed

SECTION C: PRACTICAL ASPECT IN WOUNDCARE | 165

Treatment recommendation based on the flow chart of Wound Care Algorithm:

WOUND TYPE	Wound description	Dressing material suggested/recommended (refer to chapter on dressing materials)	Antibiotic	Surgical procedure suggested/recommended
4	Wet, infected wound with < 25% slough/necrotic tissue	1. Alginate 2. Foam 3. Silver 4. Hydrofiber 5. Polymeric membrane 6. Iodine base dressing	Yes, based on C&S report of infected tissue	1. Debridement may be needed.
5	Dry, non-infected wound with >25% slough/necrotic tissue	1. Hydrogel 2. Hydrocolloid 3. Polymeric membrane	No	1. Debridement is needed
6	Wet, non-infected wound with > 25% slough/necrotic tissue	1. Alginate 2. Foam 3. Polymeric membrane 4. Hydrofiber	May or may not, based on the underlying cause.	1. Surgical/mechanical debridement is recommended. 2. May need repeated debridement

Treatment recommendation based on the flow chart of Wound Care Algorithm:

WOUND TYPE	Wound description	Dressing material suggested/recommended (refer to chapter on dressing materials)	Antibiotic	Surgical procedure suggested/recommended
7	Dry, infected wound with > 25% slough/necrotic tissue	1. Silver dressing 2. Hydrogel 3. Hydrocolloid 4. Iodine base dressing 5. Polymeric membrane	Yes, based on C&S report of infected tissue	1. Surgical/mechanical debridement is strongly recommended.
8	Wet, infected wound with > 25% slough/necrotic tissue	1. Alginate 2. Silver dressing 3. Hydrofiber 4. Foam 5. Polymeric membrane 6. charcoal 7. Iodine base dressing	Yes, based on C&S report of infected tissue	1. Surgical/mechanical debridement is strongly recommended. 2. May need repeated debridement

Appendix 1

VITAMIN AND MINERAL CONTENT IN MULTIVITAMIN TABLET (ADULT)

Vitamin/ Mineral	Dosage
Vitamin A	5000 IU
Vitamin D	400 IU
Thiamine	3.5 mg
Riboflavine	2.5 mg
Pyridoxine	2.5 mg
Cyanocobalamin	5 µg
Nicotinamide	25 mg
Ascorbic acid	50 mg
Calcium pantothenate	4 mg
Folic acid	0.5 mg
Calcium	25 mg
Copper	0.75 mg
Iron	5 mg
Iodine	0.05 mg
Manganese	0.5 mg
Magnesium	0.5 mg
Phosphorus	20 mg
Potassium	1 mg
Zinc	2 mg

1 tablet of Vitamin C = 50 mg
1 tablet of Folic Acid = 5 mg

Appendix 2

OFF-LOADING FOR DIABETIC FOOT WOUND

Introduction

Neuropathic ulcers are the prime precipitant of diabetes-related amputations of the lower extremity. The central goal of any treatment program designed to heal these wounds is effective reduction in pressure (off-loading).

Why is off-loading needed?

Elevated plantar pressure is a causative factor in the development of plantar ulcers in diabetic patients. Many structural abnormalities in a diabetic foot for an example claw toe deformity and Charcot's neuroarthropathy are among the abnormalities that can cause significant disruption to the architecture of the foot and elevate local foot pressures. Once an ulcer has formed, unless the ulcerated area is off-loaded, healing may be chronically delayed, even in an adequately perfused limb. After an ulcer is healed, the risk of recurrence is high (40% in a median of 4 months) showing the need for continuous off-loading in these patients.

Common methods to off-load the foot include;

1. Bed rest
2. Wheel chair
3. Crutch-assisted gait
4. Total contact casts
5. Felted foam
6. Removable cast walkers

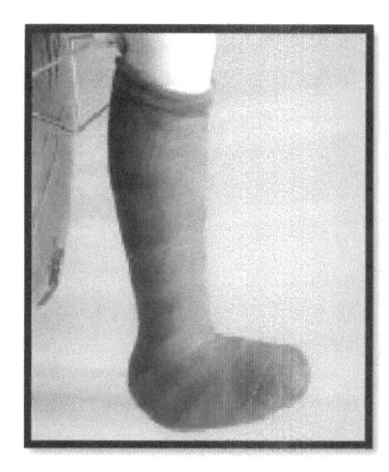

| Total contact casts | Felted foam | Removable cast |

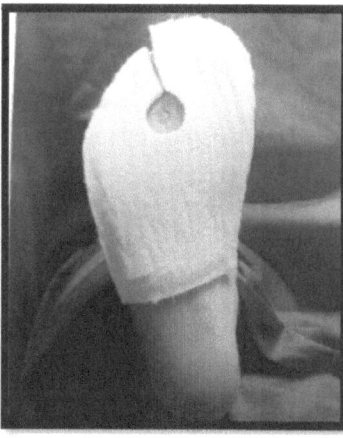

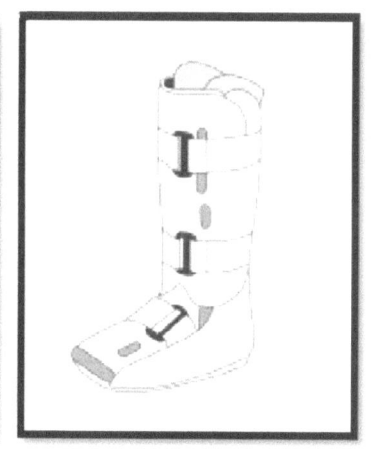

References

1. Pecoraro RE, Reiber GE, Burgess EM. Pathways to diabetic limb amputation: basis for prevention. Diabetes Care 13: 513–521, 1990

2. David G. Armstrong, DPN1234, Hienvu C. Nguyen, DPN2, Lawrence A. Lavery, DPN, MPH2, Carine H.M. van Schie, PHD3, Andrew J.M. Boulton, MD3 and Lawrence B. Harkless, DPN2. Off-Loading the Diabetic Foot Wound A randomized clinical trial

3. Wu SC, Crews RT, Armstrong DG. The pivotal role of offloading in the management of neuropathic foot ulceration. Curr Diab Rep 5:423–429, 2005.

Appendix 3

DIABETIC FOOT WEAR

Diabetic shoes, sometimes referred to as extra depth or therapeutic shoes, are specially designed shoes, or shoe inserts, intended to reduce the risk of skin breakdown in diabetics with co-existing foot disease.

When it comes to shoe selection, numerous factors need to be considered
- How long someone has had diabetes,
- Do they have normal sensation in their feet?
- Do they have any abnormalities or deformities of their feet?

Diabetic Foot Status	Type of shoes
Diabetes patients with good blood sugar control and healthy feet	Conventional shoes Patients should inspect their feet regularly
Minor foot deformities or impaired sensation and circulation	Comfort shoes, Jogging shoes, Diabetic shoes A diabetic-style shoe is characterized by being made of soft leather, has a deep toe box, has a rounder, wider toe box that can accommodate things like hammertoes and bunions

Diabetic Foot Status	Type of shoes
If foot circulation or sensation worsens or a patient develops ulcerations and significant deformities	Depth shoes combined with custom-molded inserts to redistribute pressures on the foot
Patients with extreme foot deformities	May need custom-molded shoes, in which the entire shoe is molded from a cast of the patient's foot

Tips for buying shoes

To enhance diabetic foot health, the Joslin Diabetes Center offers these tips for buying new shoes and replacing old ones:

- Buy shoes made of soft, stretchable leather.
- When possible, choose laced shoes over loafers because they fit better and offer more support.
- For better shock absorption, look for a cushioned sole instead of a thin leather sole.
- Shop for shoes later in the day because feet swell as the day progresses.
- The distance between your longest toe and the shoe tip should be half of your thumb's width.
- To ensure proper fit, try on shoes while wearing the socks that you'll be using.
- Wear new shoes for 1-2 hours for the first time, then check feet for cuts or blisters. The next day, wear them 3-4 hours and gradually build up time to make sure they aren't injuring your feet.

Replace old shoes when:

- The heel begins to collapse to one side
- The bottom of the heel is worn down
- The inner lining of the shoe is torn

Appendix 4

BRADEN SCALE FOR PREDICTING PRESSURE ULCER RISK

	1	2	3	4
Sensory Perception Ability to respond meaningfully to pressure related discomfort	**Completely Limited:** Unresponsive (does not moan, flinch, or grasp) to painful stimuli, due to diminished level of consciousness or sedation, OR Limited ability to feel pain over most of body	**Very Limited:** Responds only to painful stimuli. Cannot communicate discomfort except by moaning or restlessness, OR Has a sensory impairment, which limits the ability to feel pain or discomfort over 1/2 of body.	**Slightly Limited:** Responds to verbal commands but cannot always communicate discomfort or need to be turned, OR Has some sensory impairment, which limits ability to feel pain or discomfort in 1 or 2 extremities.	**No Impairment** Responds to verbal command. Has no sensory deficit which would limit ability to feel or voice pain or discomfort
Moisture Degree to which skin is exposed to moisture	**Constantly Moist:** Perspiration, urine, etc keep skin moist almost constantly. Dampness is detected every time patient is moved or turned.	**Moist:** Skin is often but not always moist. Linen must be changed at least once a shift.	**Occasionally Moist:** Skin is occasionally moist, requiring an extra linen change approximately once a day.	**Rarely Moist:** Skin is usually dry; linen requires changing only at routine intervals.
Activity Degree of physical activity	**Bedfast** Confined to bed	**Chairfast:** Ability to walk severely limited or nonexistent. Cannot bear own weight and/or must be assisted into chair or wheel chair.	**Walks Occasionally:** Walks occasionally during day but for very short distances, with or without assistance. Spends majority or each shift in bed or chair.	**Walks Frequently:** Walks outside the room at least twice a day and inside room at least once every 2 hours during waking hours.

	1. Completely Immobile: Does not make even slight changes in body or extremity position without assistance.	2. Very Limited: Makes occasional slight changes in body or extremity position but unable to make frequent or significant changes independently.	3. Slightly Limited: Makes frequent though slight changes in body or extremity position independently.	4. No Limitations: Makes major and frequent changes in position without assistance.	
Mobility Ability to change and control body position					
Nutrition Usual food intake pattern	1. Very Poor: Never eats a complete meal. Rarely eats more than 1/3 of any food offered.	2. Probably Inadequate Rarely eats a complete meal And generally eats only about ½ of any food offered. Protein intake Includes only 3 servings of meat or dairy products per day. Occasionally will take a dietary supplement, OR Receives less than optimum amount of liquid diet or tube feeding.	3. Adequate: Eats over half of most meals. Eats a total of 4 servings of protein (meat, dairy products) each day. Occasionally will refuse a meal, but will usually take a supplement if offered, OR Is on a tube feeding or TPN regimen, which probably meets most of nutritional needs.	4. Excellent: Eats most of every meal. Never refuses a meal. Usually eats a total of 4 or more servings of meat and dairy products. Occasionally eats between meals. Does not require supplementation.	
Friction and Shear	1. Problem: Requires moderate to maximum assistance in moving. Complete lifting without sliding against sheets is impossible. Frequently slides down in bed or chair, requiring frequent repositioning with maximum assistance. Spasticity, contractures, or agitation leads to almost constant friction.	2. Potential Problem: Moves feebly or requires minimum assistance. During a move skin probably slides to some extent against sheets, chair, restraints, or other devices. Maintains relatively good position in chair or bed most of the time but occasionally slides down	3. No Apparent Problem: Moves in bed and in chair independently and has sufficient muscle strength to lift up completely during move. Maintains good position in bed or chair at all times.		
					Total Score

- *Generally not at risk:* *(Braden score: 19-23)*
- *At risk:* *(Braden score: 15-18)*
- *Moderate risk:* *(Braden score: 13-14)*
- *High risk:* *(Braden score: 10-12)*
- *Very high risk:* *(Braden score: ≤9)*

Note: When Braden scale score is 16 or less, implement pressure ulcer prevention measures

Pressure Ulcer Prevention Measures (to be implemented when Braden scale score is 16 or less)

May be used as a guide and may adjust to suit local setting

	STAFF APPROACHES/IMPLEMENTATION
Pressure relieving method	Implement a turning schedule e.g. 2-hourly turning
	When side-lying position is used a 30 degree turning position should be used. Avoid positioning directly on trochanter.
	Keep head of bed in lowest degree of elevation consistent with medical condition (optimum is less than 30 degrees except at mealtime).
	Place pressure reduction device on the bed, chair or wheelchair
	Use device such as pillows or foam wedges to prevent direct contact between bony prominences
	Use lift sheet
	Use heels and elbow protector
	DO NOT use donut device
	Encourage patient to shift their weight every 15 minute for 15 seconds while on a wheelchair. (Recommended for paraplegic patient with sensory loss)

Skin care	Inspect skin at least once/day
	Individualize bathing schedule
	Use lubricants to reduce friction injuries; moisturizers for dry skin
	Cleanse skin at time of soiling and PRN
	Use protective barrier on skin
Bowel and bladder care	Evaluate and manage urinary and/or fecal incontinence., consider colostomy and CBD for selected cases
Others	Consult PT/OT regarding mobility needs as indicated.
	Provide ROM exercise BID
	Consult dietician to assist with nutritional assessment and planning
	Provide patient education materials as indicated

Appendix 5

PAIN SCALES

Visual Analogue Score (VAS)

This is a 100 mm line indicating two extremes for no pain and worst pain. Patients are asked to point to a position the line that best indicates their level of pain which is then measured and recorded.

Numerical Rating scales (NRS)

The patient is asked to rate the pain on a scale of 0-10 where 0 (zero) is "no pain at all" and 10 (ten) is "the worst pain imaginable"
In the Ministry of Health hospitals, we use a combination of the two scales where the patient is shown a ruler with numbers (1 to 10) and a slider to indicate the level of his/her pain.

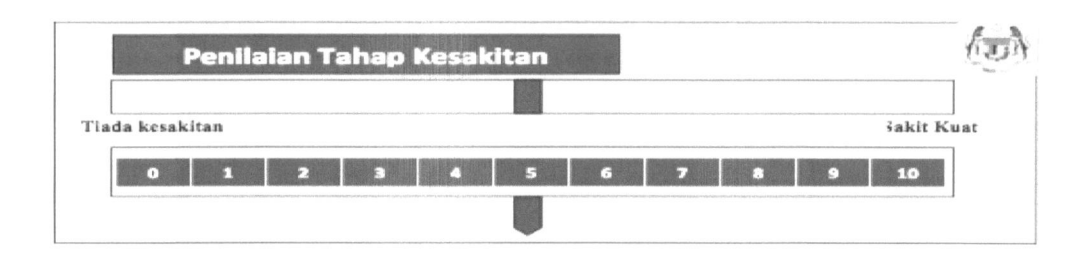

Faces scale, used for children aged 1-4 years, uses cartoon faces ranging from a smiling face to a tearful face.
The patient is asked to indicate the face that best represents his/her pain level. The number on the face is multiplied by two to get a score out of 10.

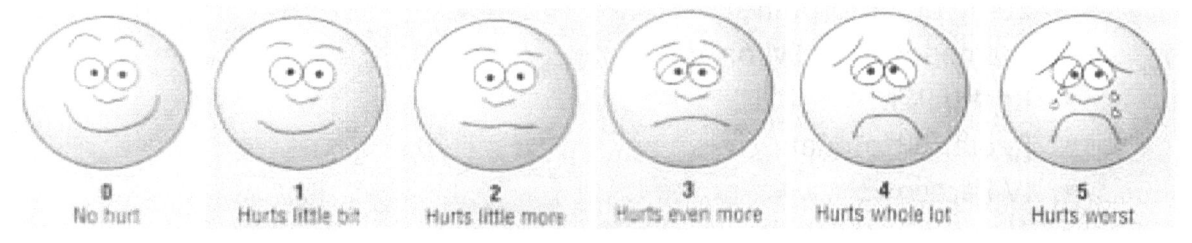

The Wong-Baker faces scale (adapted from Wong DL. et al., eds. Whaley and Wong's essentials of pediatric nursing. 5th ed. St Louis, MO: Mosby, 2001)

Appendix 6

ANALGESIC LADDER FOR ACUTE PAIN MANAGEMENT

Analgesic Ladder for Acute Pain Management

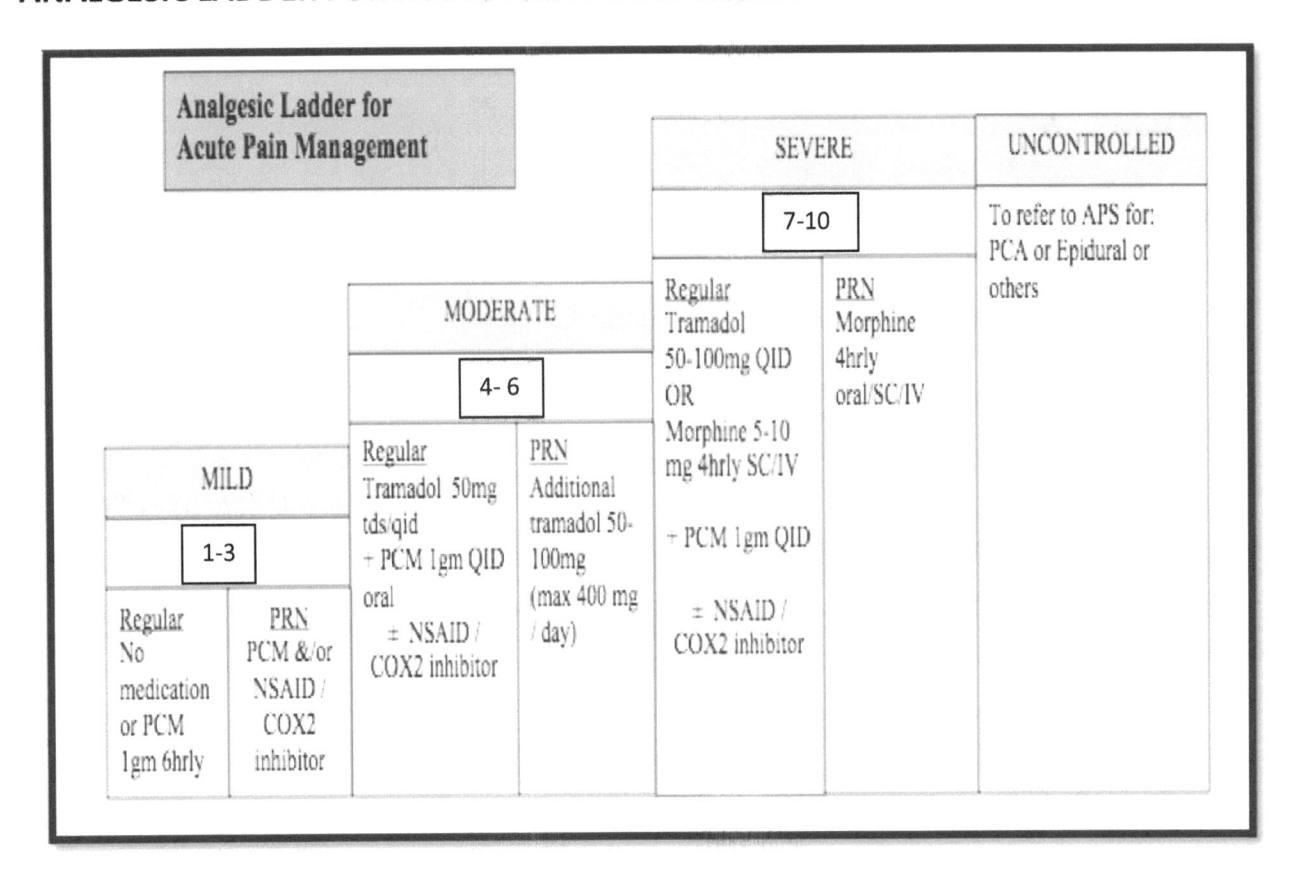

MILD (1-3)	MODERATE (4-6)	SEVERE (7-10)	UNCONTROLLED
Regular: No medication or PCM 1gm 6hrly	Regular Tramadol 50mg tds/qid + PCM 1gm QID oral ± NSAID / COX2 inhibitor	Regular Tramadol 50-100mg QID OR Morphine 5-10 mg 4hrly SC/IV + PCM 1gm QID ± NSAID / COX2 inhibitor	To refer to APS for: PCA or Epidural or others
PRN: PCM &/or NSAID / COX2 inhibitor	PRN Additional tramadol 50-100mg (max 400 mg / day)	PRN Morphine 4hrly oral/SC/IV	

NOTES:

1. Weak opioids include DF118 and tramadol.

2. In NBM patients oral drugs may be replaced by any of any of the following, depending of the pain level.

- Morphine SC or IV (Note that 10mg IV morphine is equivalent to 20mg oral morphine)
- Tramadol SC or IM or IV
- Rectal PCM
- Rectal Diclofenac
- IV Parecoxib

- NSAIDs are contraindicated in patients with hypovolemia, peptic ulcer disease and history of allergy to aspirin or other NSAIDs. They should be used with caution in patients with thrombocytopenia, coagulopathies and asthma, as well as in patients with renal, hepatic or cardiac impairment. Avoid in the elderly (>65yrs), or if necessary, use a lower dose of NSAID. For those at risk of peptic ulcer or gastritis, add a Proton Pump Inhibitor or use COX2 inhibitors instead of NSAIDs.

- For those in severe pain, use SC or IV morphine and titrate to comfort (See Morphine Pain Protocol, *Appendix 9*)

Appendix 7

FORMULATIONS AND DOSAGE OF COMMONLY USED ANALGESICS

DRUG	FORMULATION AVAILABLE	DOSAGE
Paracetamol	Tablet 500mg, Suspension 500mg/5ml, Suppositories	500 mg – 1gm qid
NSAIDs		
Diclofenac	Tablet 50mg & 25mg, IM injections Suppositories 12.5mg, 25mg, (50mg & 100mg)* Gel	Oral 25 - 50mg tds, (max 3 doses/day) IM 25-50mgs tds (max 3doses/day) (not encouraged) Sup: 50mg-100mg stat Topical: PRN
Mefenamic Acid (Ponstan)	Capsule 250mg	250 mg – 500mg tds
Ibuprofen (Brufen)	Tablet 200mg & 400mg*	200 mg – 400 mg tds
Naproxen (Naprosyn, Synflex)	Tablet 250mg, 550mg	500mg-550 mg bd
Ketoprofen (Orudis, Oruvail)	Capsule 100mg *, Injection 100mg, Patch 30mg, Gel	Oral: 100mg daily, IV: 100mg bd Patch: 30mg - 60mg bd, Topical: PRN
Meloxicam (Mobic)	Tab 7.5mg	Daily or bd
COX 2 inhibitors		
Celecoxib	Capsule 200 mg, 400mg	200 mg bd /400mg OD (max 1 week)
Etoricoxib	Tablet 90 mg & 120 mg	120 mg daily (max 1 week)
Parecoxib	Injection 20 mg/ml	40 mg bd (20 mg bd for elderly) max for 2 days
WEAK OPIOIDs		
Tramadol	Capsule 50mg, Injection 50mg/ml	50mg -100mg tds or qid (max 400mg/day) IM not encouraged

Dihydrocodeine (DF118)	Tablet 30 mg	30mg-60mg qid (max 360mg/day)
STRONG OPIOIDs		
Morphine (1st line)	Tablet SR 10mg, 30mg Aqueous 10mg / 5ml Injection 10 mg/ml,	SR morphine for severe background pain Aq morphine to be given at least 30 minutes prior to procedure Inj - to be given Subcut. 30 minutes prior to procedure Dosage: # < 60yrs : 5mg -10mg > 60yrs : 2.5mg -5mg
Oxycodone	Tablet SR Oxycontin, 10mg, 20mg Immediate release – Capsule. Oxynorm 5mg, 10 mg	SR Oxycontin 10-20mg bd for severe background pain IR oxynorm 5-10mg 4 hrly
Pethidine Use of pethidine is not encouraged due to the risk of norpethidine toxicity and higher addiction potential.	Injection 50mg/ml 100mg/2ml	IV/ IM / SC <60 yrs 50mg-100 mg 4hrly >60yrs 25mg-50mg 4hrly Reduce dose in renal and hepatic impairment
Fentanyl FOR APS USE ONLY	Injection 50 mcg/ml, Patch 25 mcg/h, 50 mcg/h	IV only to be prescribed by APS team. Patch to be used for severe background pain in cancer pain; NOT in Acute Pain

Appendix 8

SEDATION SCORE

0 = none (patient is alert)
1 = mild (patient is sometimes drowsy)
2 = moderate (patient is often drowsy but easily arousable)
3 = unarousable
S = patient is asleep, easily arousable

Respiratory Depression

Respiratory depression may occur with overdose of opioids.
However, it is always associated with sedation; in fact, if patient has a sedation score of 3 (unarousable) without a decrease in the respiratory rate, this is considered as an overdose of opioid.
The risk of respiratory depression is minimal if strong opioids are titrated to effect and only used to relieve pain (i.e. not to help patients to sleep or to calm down agitated patients).
The risk of respiratory depression is also minimal in patients on chronic opioid use (e.g. patients on morphine for cancer pain).

Diagnosis of Respiratory Depression

- Respiratory Rate <8/min AND Sedation Score = 2 (difficult to arouse) OR
- Sedation Score = 3 (unarousable)

To confirm opioid-induced respiratory depression – check pupils (will be pin-point if this is due to opioid overdose)

Management

- Administer oxygen – face mask or nasal prongs
- Stimulate the patient – tell him/her to breathe
- Dilute Naloxone 0.4 mg / ml in 4 mls water or normal saline. Administer Naloxone 0.1 mg (1 ml) every 1-2 minutes until the patient wakes up or respiratory rate is more than 10/minute.
- Continue to monitor the respiratory rate and sedation score every hourly for at least another 4 hours. If respiratory depression or oversedation recurs, a second dose of naloxone may be required. After treating with the second dose of naloxone, you should refer the patient

to the ICU or HDU for close monitoring as the patient may require a naloxone infusion.

Naloxone

Naloxone is a pure opioid antagonist.
It is available in ampoules of 0.4 mg/ml (adult dose) or 0.02 mg/ml (paediatric dose).

Doses for treating opioid-induced respiratory depression:

- Adult 0.1 – 0.4 mg IV/IM/SC; IV dose may be repeated every 1-2 minutes
- Paediatric 0.01 mg/kg IV (maximum 0.4 mg), repeat every 2 minutes.

The half life of naloxone is 45-60 minutes; this is important to know because when used to antagonize respiratory depression due to morphine, the effect of naloxone may wear out before the effect of morphine (half life 3-4 hours). Therefore, after treating morphine-induced respiratory depression, the patient has to be monitored closely for at least another 4 hours. Naloxone should be available in every emergency drug trolley.

Appendix 9

MORPHINE PROTOCOL FOR DOCTORS

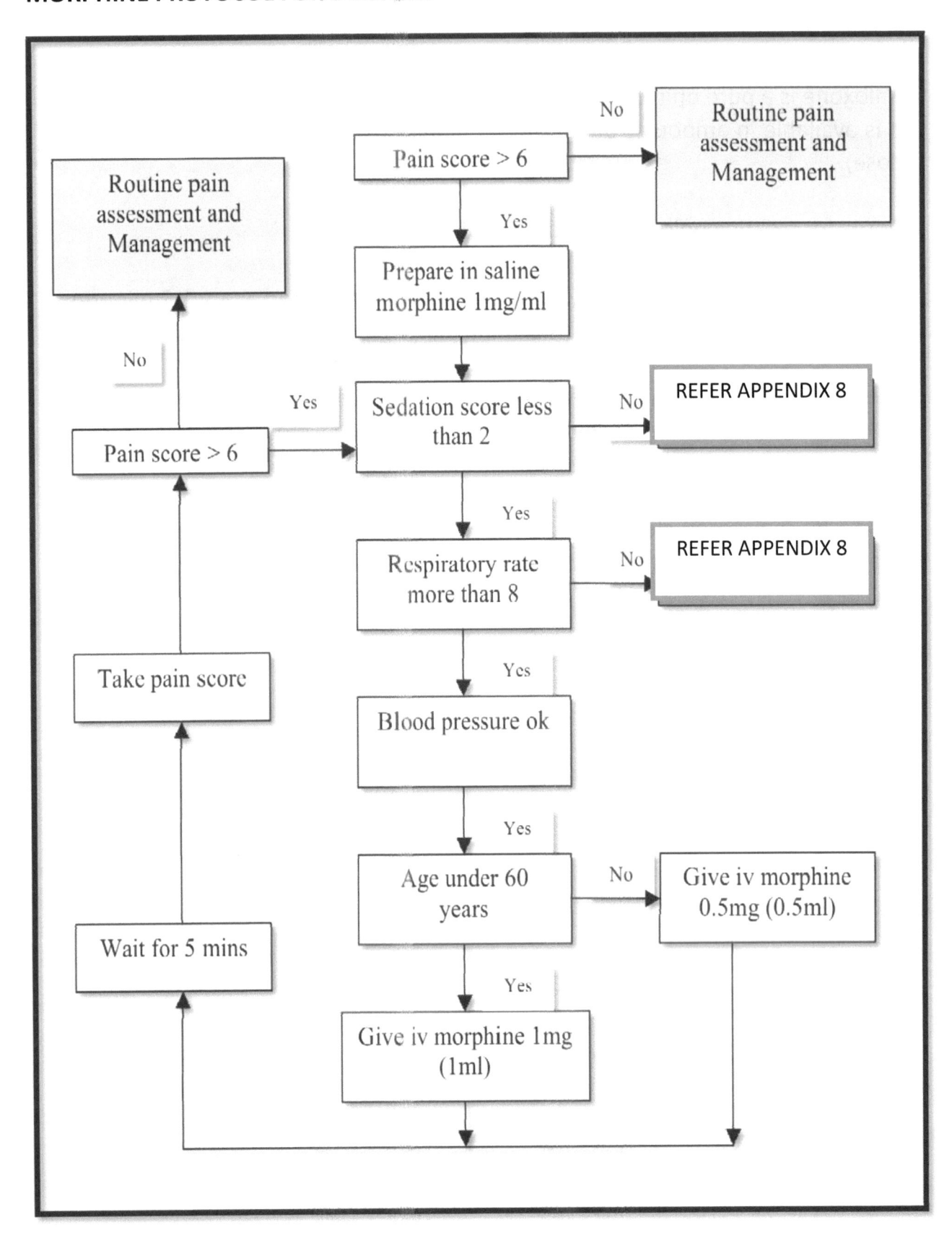

```
                                    ┌─── No ──→ Routine pain
                    Pain score > 6 ─┤           assessment and
                          │ Yes                 Management
                          ↓
                    Prepare in saline
                    morphine 1mg/ml
                          │
   Routine pain           ↓
   assessment and   ┌─── Sedation score less ─── No ──→ REFER APPENDIX 8
   Management       │    than 2
         ↑          │ Yes
         │ No       ↓
   Pain score > 6 ──┘
         ↑          Respiratory rate ─── No ──→ REFER APPENDIX 8
         │          more than 8
   Take pain score        │ Yes
         ↑                ↓
         │          Blood pressure ok
   Wait for 5 mins        │ Yes
         ↑                ↓
         │          Age under 60 ─── No ──→ Give iv morphine
         │          years                    0.5mg (0.5ml)
         │                │ Yes
         │                ↓
         │          Give iv morphine 1mg
         │          (1ml)
         └────────────────┘
```

APPENDIX | 184

Appendix 10

MORPHINE PAIN PROTOCOL FOR TRAINED (ACCREDITED) PARAMEDICS

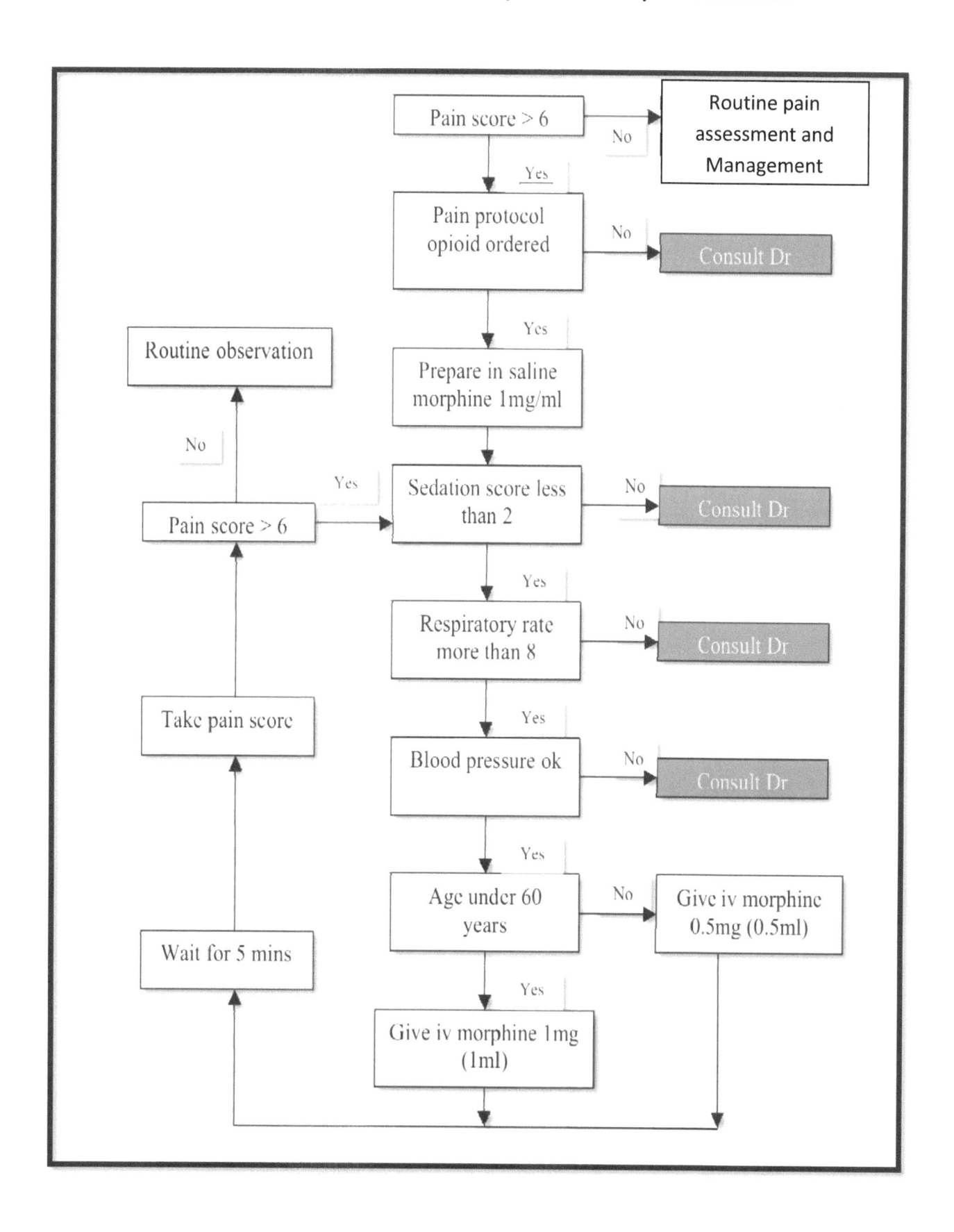

```
                                    Pain score > 6 ──No──▶ Routine pain
                                          │                assessment and
                                         Yes               Management
                                          ▼
                                    Pain protocol ──No──▶ Consult Dr
                                    opioid ordered
                                          │
                                         Yes
                                          ▼
    Routine observation            Prepare in saline
            ▲                      morphine 1mg/ml
            │No                           │
            │                             ▼
    Pain score > 6 ──Yes──▶ Sedation score less ──No──▶ Consult Dr
            ▲                    than 2
            │                       │
            │                      Yes
            │                       ▼
    Take pain score            Respiratory rate ──No──▶ Consult Dr
            ▲                  more than 8
            │                       │
            │                      Yes
            │                       ▼
            │                  Blood pressure ok ──No──▶ Consult Dr
            │                       │
            │                      Yes
            │                       ▼
    Wait for 5 mins            Age under 60 ──No──▶ Give iv morphine
            ▲                  years                0.5mg (0.5ml)
            │                       │
            │                      Yes
            │                       ▼
            │                  Give iv morphine 1mg
            │                  (1ml)
            │                       │
            └───────────────────────┴──────────────────────┘
```